हठयोगप्रदीपिका

Haṭha Yoga Pradīpīkā

हठयोगप्रदीपिका

Haṭha Yoga Pradīpīkā

The Classic Guide for the Advanced Practice of Haṭha Yoga

YOGI SVATMARAMA

Containing
The Practical Commentary of Swami Vishnudevananda
Founder of International Sivananda Yoga Vedanta Centre

MOTILAL BANARSIDASS PUBLISHERS
PRIVATE LIMITED • DELHI
SIVANANDA YOGA VEDANTA CENTRE

Reprint: Delhi, 2016
Second Revised Edition: Delhi, 2008
First Indian Edition: Delhi 1999
First Published: Canada, 1987

In Association With
SIVANANDA YOGA VEDANTA CENTRE
8th Avenue, Val Morin, Queber, JoT 2RO Canada
Tel: 819 3223 226
Email: hq@sivananda.org
www.sivananda.org

ISBN: 978-81-208-1614-5

MOTILAL BANARSIDASS

41 U.A. Bungalow Road, Jawahar Nagar, Delhi 110 007
8 Mahalaxmi Chamber, 22 Bhulabhai Desai Road, Mumbai 400 026
203 Royapettah High Road, Mylapore, Chennai 600 004
236, 9th Main III Block, Jayanagar, Bengaluru 560 011
8 Camac Street, Kolkata 700 017
Ashok Rajpath, Patna 800 004
Chowk, Varanasi 221 001

Printed in India

by RP Jain at NAB Printing Unit,
A-44, Naraina Industrial Area, Phase I, New Delhi–110028
and published by JP Jain for Motilal Banarsidass Publishers (P) Ltd,
41 U.A. Bungalow Road, Jawahar Nagar, Delhi-110007

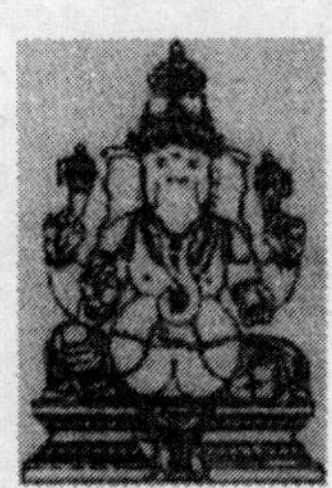

TABLE OF CONTENTS

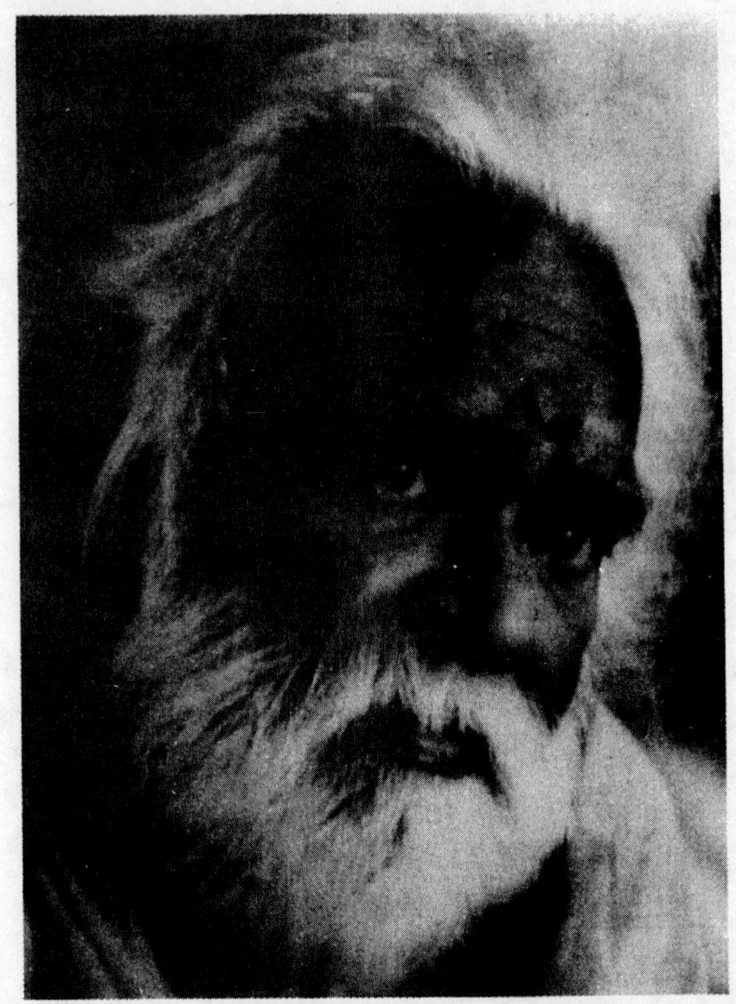

Swami Vishnudevananda (1927-1993)

PREFACE

When the Executive Board Members of the Sivananda Yoga Vedanta Centre expressed an interest to re-issue the renowned Hatha Yoga treatise, the *Haṭha Yoga Pradīpīkā,* I was very pleased to offer my services in this regard. The result is a revision of the 1987 edition which retains the original Commentary and Introduction of Swami Vishnudevananda. Please note that Swami Vishnudevananda's teachings were mainly oral and the commentary in the book is based on his talks given to students. We have preserved the original style of his delivery. I would like to thank the Sivananda Yoga Vedanta Centre for giving me this opportunity to serve and offer this work as a simple gift to Swami Vishnudevananda and his mission to create peace in the world.

S. Rajaman
Montreal, Canada
2008

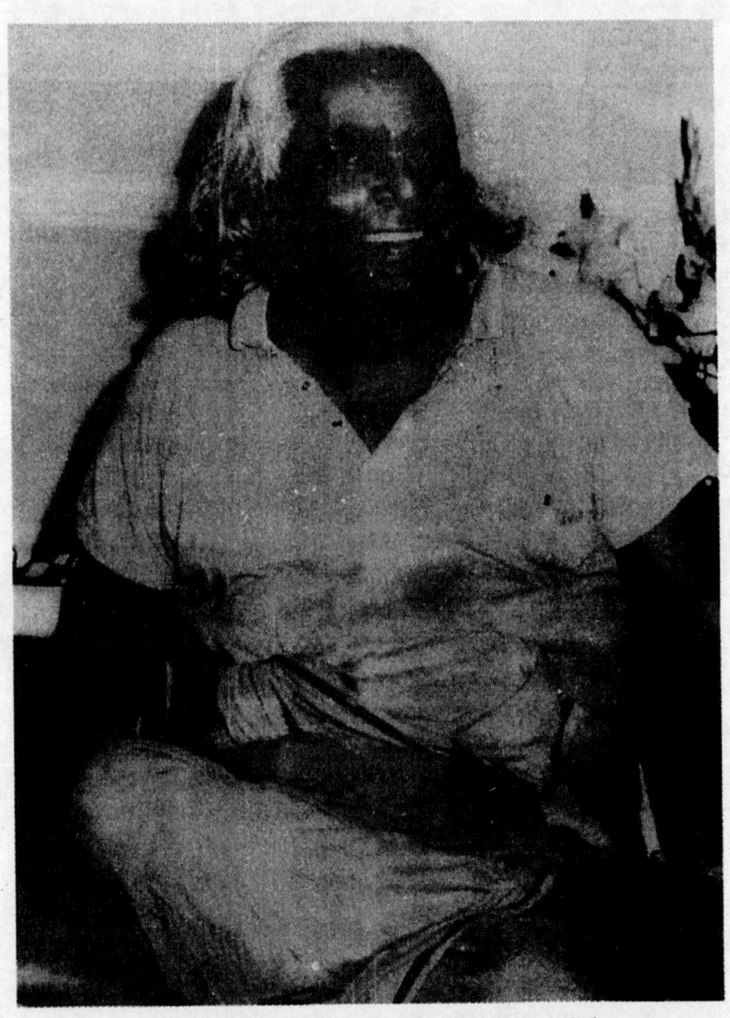

*Published in honour of the 60th Birthday
"Diamond Jubilee Celebration"
of Swami Vishnudevananda
by his disciples and devotees*

INTRODUCTION BY SWAMI VISHNUDEVANANDA TO THE 1987 TRANSLATION

I would like to begin by speaking about the spiritual path we are climbing through Yoga. You might say that it is an uphill climb. There are ups and downs. We climb up and then once again go down. There is no straight path to the top and there are many obstacles. In some places the road is wide but then suddenly it narrows. We come to a bush through which it is very difficult to penetrate, and even though we continue, we do not know where we are going.

So it is with the spiritual journey. In the beginning it is all very wonderful: "Ah, yes, I can do asanas, pranayama, etc.", but then suddenly you come to that big bush in your path and you don't know in which direction to go. If somehow you come out of the bush, you come next to a swamp. Some students disappear in the quicksand and never come out. Perhaps they see a beautiful girl or a handsome man and get married, and oh, they want to enjoy their life with children, home and family - once again swallowed by Maya, their spiritual purpose completely forgotten.

Nevertheless, it is possible to penetrate these obstacles and reach the top. Now you can see all around beautifully. Now you can meditate and enjoy full freedom. No more birth, no more death; you've got an eternal holiday.

These experiences are familiar to the yogi. He finds no smooth road to the top. Those who succeed come from different directions, having followed different teachers, but once they reach the top, everything is the same. On the way the obstacles will differ, but at the top the view is the same.

The purpose of the practice of Yoga is to give your life a boost, to put your spiritual progress in first gear. Then you may go into second gear and maybe into third gear where you can cruise comfortably after climbing the hills. This is unlike most worldly people who just coast downhill without knowing about brakes, thinking that happiness is somewhere down there, waiting. They go straight downhill, faster and faster into numerous disasters such as cancer, AIDS, high blood pressure, heart trouble. Soon it is too late and they crash. So even though it may seem very easy, please don't coast downhill. We will show you another way.

The path was laid out by the *Hatha Yoga Pradīpikā*, an ancient text used by Yogis to create the power to go uphill all the way to the top. This path was laid out by great beings called siddhas: Matsyendranath, his disciple Gorakshanath and others, fourteen in all. This is one of the earliest treatises on Hatha Yoga; all the modern books are based on it. It is the central route. All of us have only expanded and expounded on it in different ways.

In addition to following the practices laid out in the *Hatha Yoga Pradīpikā*, I strongly recommend the study of books such as Shankaracharya's *Viveka Chudamani*, and the *Srimad Bhagavatam*. The *Viveka Chudamani* is a very beautiful book, and those who follow its instruction will create the necessary dispassion to surmount the obstacles created by rajas (passion or activity). In addition, we also need devotion, because without God's grace we cannot reach the Source no matter how hard we strive. To help create this devotion, we read from the Bhagavatam.

This practice is not something I invented; it is the traditional method which I myself followed intensively when I was with Master Sivananda in the Himalayas. I lived in the forest where there were cobras and tigers. Sometimes I could hear the tigers from my cottage when they would come by to drink water and they would roar. I had only a flimsy door which they could easily have pushed through. Nevertheless, in such an environment I went through this training morning, noon, evening and midnight, practicing for almost fourteen hours daily. I hardly slept - just two or three hours a night. But I can't begin to describe the power that builds up.

Our purpose here is to increase the vibratory level in a very short time. In Sanskrit this work is expressed as "Shakti Sanchar." Shakti is the "power" and Sanchar means "awakening of." We want to make the Shakti move from its dormant or static state to the dynamic state through sadhana or spiritual practice. However, please be careful not to go beyond your capacity. Do not do too much at once, do not go too deep or too fast, do not work too intensively, or else a kickback will come. That is why I modify the practice to suit the particular evolution of my students. I never give a practice unless I myself have experienced it. Also, though I like discipline, I believe that this discipline must come from within. I show my students how this can be accomplished and then leave them to practice as if they were alone in the forest. To this is added just a little group practice for reinforcement. In addition, my students make out a resolve form and keep a spiritual diary which I look at to check their progress so that I can prescribe a little more or a little less of a particular practice. We meet together for an hour each day to talk about our practice, to receive some instruction about technical things and to improve the performance of some of these procedures.

My main instruction is to control the mind. Secondly, avoid unnecessary desires with one exception - desire to increase your will power. If you satisfy one desire, ten more will come to take its place, and then when will you ever be finished with all those desires? But if you develop your will power and kill even one desire, then you will be strong. Then you will easily kill ten more, and then a hundred.

Om Namah Sivaya!

Swami Vishnudevananda

Publisher's Note

This book is intended as an aid for those who wish to learn the advanced practices of Hatha Yoga from a qualified teacher. It is suggested that it also be used in conjunction with the *Complete Illustrated Book of Yoga* by Swami Vishnudevananda, the *Sivananda Companion to Yoga* (the *New Book of Yoga*), and *Yoga Mind and Body* both by the Sivananda Yoga Vedanta Centre.

Many of the instructions given here have been purposely veiled by the original writers, others need elaboration, and many require the guidance of a teacher. Swami Vishnudevananda repeatedly stressed that these practices are not for beginners, and that to violate this caution is to put the psyche at risk. Please therefore, follow the instructions along with the guidance of your guru.

Sivananda Yoga Vedanta Centre
Val Morin, Quebec, Canada
2008

हठयोगप्रदीपिका
Haṭha Yoga Pradīpīkā
CHAPTER ONE

श्रीआदिनाथ नमोऽस्तु तस्मै येनोपदिष्टा हठयोगविद्या।
विभ्राजते   प्रोन्नतराजयोगमारोदुमिच्छोरधिरोहिणीव ॥ १ ॥

(1) Maṅgala śloka: Salutations to the primeval Being (Lord Śiva) who is the instructor of the Haṭhayoga-Vidyā (to Pārvatī), which shines bright like a ladder for one desirous to climb to the heights of the most excellent Rājayoga.

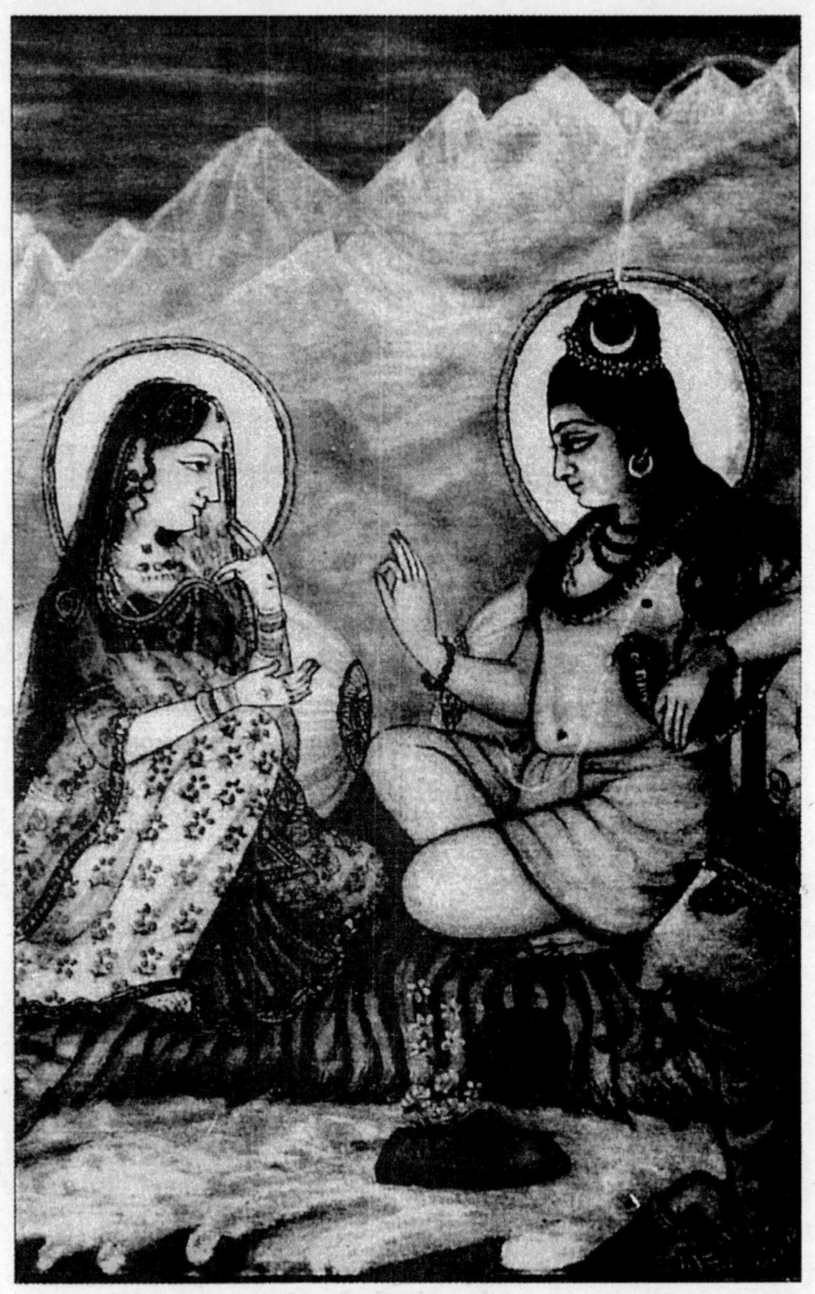

श्रीआदिनाथ नमोऽस्तु तस्मै येनोपदिष्टा हठयोगविद्या।
विभ्राजते   प्रोन्नतराजयोगमारोढुमिच्छोरधिरोहिणीव ॥ १ ॥

(1) Maṅgala śloka: Salutations to the primeval Being (Lord Śiva) who is the instructor of the Haṭhayoga-Vidyā (to Pārvatī), which shines bright like a ladder for one desirous to climb to the heights of the most excellent Rājayoga.

Svatmarama begins the teaching in the traditional way, by prostrating before the gurus. First he prostrates before the Adi Guru, the first guru — Lord Siva, and then before his disciple Matsyendranath and his disciple Gorakshanath. Through their grace, Svatmarama expounds this great science.

Vidya means knowledge. The knowledge of Hatha Yoga was first taught by Siva to his consort Parvati, the Universal Mother.

The purpose of Hatha Yoga is to give you the knowledge of controlling these two energies "Ha" and "Tha" (Prana and Apana). Without this knowledge it is very difficult to gain that control over the mind, which is called Raja Yoga. Raja Yoga deals with the mind, Hatha Yoga works with the prana and apana. Many students make the mistake of considering Hatha Yoga to be mainly asanas, when actually asana is only one of the eight steps of Hatha Yoga. Furthermore, there is no real difference between Hatha Yoga and Raja Yoga. There is no possibility of attaining Raja Yoga without the practice of Hatha Yoga, and vice versa. Hatha Yoga is the practical way to control the mind through control of the prana.

Look at the fluttering of the leaves on a tree. By watching this fluttering you can infer the speed of the wind, even though you cannot see the wind itself. In the same way, we cannot see the prana or the apana, or the motion of the mind or its thoughts. According to Raja Yoga, mind is like a lake, and thought the waves (or vrittis in Sanskrit). Raja Yoga is controlling and eventually stopping these waves of thought. In Sanskrit we say, "Yoga chitta vritti nirodha."

According to Patanjali, author of the [Raja] Yoga Sutras, there are five kinds of vrittis, some being positive and some not. Of these five, only one is entirely positive, and that is when the seer identifies with the Self (the Atman). This is only possible when the thought waves are slowed down. Then the seer sees, in the calm lake of the mind, his own Self (Atman). But as long as the wind exists, we will see the tree moving, the leaves fluttering - sometimes quietly sometimes violently, but always moving.

Hatha Yoga asks, "How do you stop these waves?" and "How does the seer see the Self?"

As the waves on the lake are created by the wind on the lake, so also the waves on the mind are created by the prana and apana. Sometimes this energy moves very fast, sometimes slow. And according to the nature of the prana/apana motion, the thought waves will be very intense or very slow. We call this rajasic or tamasic thought.

Tamasic waves are lethargic and sleepy, for then inertia prevails. It is not a still, peaceful state of mind, or an active state of mind; it is an inert state, where mind is incapable of doing anything. It just vegetates like a stone or a block of ice. Tamasic waves are very dull and gross, frozen like ice, so that you can't see your reflection even though the surface seems to be still. It is impossible to see what's at the bottom of the lake.

Rajasic waves are like a stormy sky. It is agitated. Waves arise on the lake, arise and dissolve continuously on the turbulent surface of the mind.

But in the sattvic state, the waves become still; there is no motion of the prana apana because the energy has been diverted to the central channel, the Sushumna. Ordinarily, when these waves are projected, the prana/apana moves through the Ida and Pingala channels on the right and left sides of the body. This can be demonstrated by checking your brain waves.

Sometimes the right hemisphere is more active; sometimes it is the left that is more active. Waves from the left hemisphere are mostly analytical, mathematical, scientific, rational, etc. Generally, these are the waves most used by the Western mind. That is why you (in the West) have created beautiful cities and cars and complex technologies. It is because your left hemisphere most often dominates the right hemisphere. Even your religions emphasize the left, analytical side. When Christian monks go into seclusion, they indulge in contemplation rather than in meditation, and in Judaism, the usual rabbinical approach to religion is analytical.

Waves coming from the right brain are philosophical, devotional, compassionate, peaceful in nature, even though we use them mostly for inertia or for emotional things. Either you love or you have somebody, and so you put the waves on a very gross or tamasic level.

The purpose of Yoga is to prevent either hemisphere from dominating the other, to create the sattvic state. That is why we meditate in a place where there is very little activity - just the simple natural motion of the trees in the breeze and occasionally the calls of some birds. In our ashrams we plant flowers. All this is to help calm the mind.

The main practice of Yoga is to the left side of the brain by using the right brain. When the left brain is active, Ida is functioning and breath is moving through the right nostril. When the right brain is operating, the left nostril is opened and Pingala is functioning. Normally this changes every one and a half to two hours. alternating back and forth. But when the energy is not moving through either the left or right nadi, it must go through the Sushumna, and then the energy is balanced.

Moreover, the awareness of time and space is caused by this motion of waves of prana between the right and left channels. There is some similarity between samadhi and deep sleep. In deep sleep you are not aware of time or space because the vrittis are suppressed: they are not stopped as in samadhi. You might say that in deep sleep the vrittis are on ice - in cold storage. They will come back when the sun comes up to melt the ice. But in samadhi there are no vrittis at all. Ordinarily the only time we experience such quiet is during deep sleep, a state of inertia, but in samadhi the mental modifications have been suspended. Then there is balance between the right and left brains. For this we practice alternate nostril breathing because we can't directly affect the brain itself.

प्रणम्य श्रीगुरुं नाथं स्वात्मारामेण योगिना।
केवलं राजयोगाय हठविद्योपदिश्यते ॥ २ ॥

*(2) Bowing to his respected guru, Yogī Svātmārāma
gives instruction on Haṭhayoga for the sole purpose of
achieving Rājayoga.*

Following tradition, he first salutes his own guru in order to get the
benefit of the teaching. You must salute your teacher because God
is manifesting the teaching through him. Here it is Siva who is
manifesting through Svatmarama's teacher.

Raja Yoga means control of thought waves, something which is not
possible without Hatha Yoga. Svatmarama is not talking about
asana or even about the physical breathing, but about the subtle
current which creates the thought waves.

भ्रान्त्या   बहुमतध्वान्ते राजयोगमजानताम् ।
हठीप्रदीपिकां धत्ते स्वात्मारामः कृपाकरः ॥ ३ ॥

*(3) Svātmārāma, the compassionate one, has
composed the Haṭhayoga-pradīpīkā for the sake of
those who do not know (are unacquainted with)
Rājayoga, because of the confusion generated in the
form of the darkness of the presence of conflicting
ideas.*

You can translate the words "Raja Yoga" here to mean control of
thought currents. Those who are unable to obtain Raja Yoga are
those who are still unable to control their own thought when they
meditate; their thoughts continue to come up. The aim of Raja Yoga
is to stop the thought waves, but when you cannot do that, you try
to lean to control the prana. In order to control the prana, you
control the physical breath. In this way, through the physical you
go to the subtle prana, and then to an even subtler level - to
thoughts. As they are all interrelated, one affects the other.

What does he mean by "conflicting sects?" Someone will say to do
this, another will say to repeat mantras or to do that. Hatha Yoga
is a scientific approach to subduing the thought current by
subduing the prana. That is accomplished when there are no
waves. The seer sees Himself, the seer and the seen become one. The

seer identifies with the Self. In this state there are no vrittis (thoughts waves). It is something like looking at the bright light of the sun or the high beam of an approaching car. After some time you are blinded. When the vrittis subside as a result of doing pranayama, that is called Raja Yoga. That state is the seer seeing the Self.

The "light of Hatha Vidya" is the knowledge of Hatha Yoga.

हठविद्यां   हि मत्स्येन्द्रगोरक्षाद्या विजानते।
स्वात्मारामोऽथवा योगी जानीते तत्प्रसादतः ॥ ४ ॥

(4) Matsyendra, Gorakṣa, and others are great adepts of Haṭhavidyā. Yogī Svātmārāma has come to possess the science of Haṭhayoga by the grace and blessings of these great savants.

This is the beginning of an account of the lineage of those who received this knowledge. According to tradition, through the grace of Lord Siva, Yogi Matsyendra was a fish who was changed into a human being and received the Hatha Vidya from Lord Siva himself. Knowledge does not come from just anywhere. It is like milk, which comes only from the udders of a cow. You cannot milk the ear. It is the same with the guru. Knowledge may be everywhere, but you cannot get the knowledge from anywhere except through the guru-disciple lineage. So Siva Gorakshanath, and through their grace eventually Svatmarama the author of this book learned Hatha Yoga. In Sanskrit this is called "guruparampara."

श्रीआदिनाथमत्स्येन्द्रशबरानन्दभैरवाः ।
चौरङ्गीमीनगोरक्षविरूपाक्षविलेशया: ॥ ५ ॥

(5) Lord Śiva, Matsyendra, Śābara, Ānandabhairava, Cauraṅgī, Mīna, Gorakṣa, Virūpākṣa, Bileśaya.

मन्थानो भैरवो योगी सिद्धिर्बुद्धश्च कन्थडिः ।
कोरण्टकः सुरानन्दः सिद्धिपादश्च चर्पटिः ॥ ६ ॥

(6) Manthāna, Bhairava yogī, Siddhi, Buddha, Kanthaḍi, Korantaka, Surānanda, Siddhapāda, Carpaṭi.

कानेरी   पूज्यपादश्च   नित्यनाथो निरञ्जन: ।
कपाली बिन्दुनाथश्च काकचण्डीश्वाराह्वय: ॥ ७ ॥

(7) Kānerī, Pūjyapāda, Nityanātha, Nirañjana, Kapālī, Bindunātha, Kākacaṇḍīśvara.

अल्लाम: प्रभुदेवश्च घोडाचोली च टिण्टिणि: ।
भानुकी नारदेवश्च खण्ड: कापालिकस्तथा ॥ ८ ॥

(8) Allāma, Prabhudeva, Ghoḍācolī, Ṭiṇṭiṇi, Bhānukī, Nāradeva, Khaṇḍa, Kāpālika.

इत्यादयो   महासिद्धा   हठयोगप्रभावत: ।
खण्डयित्वा कालदण्डं ब्रह्माण्डे विचरन्ति ते ॥ ९ ॥

(9) The above mentioned are great siddhas due to their prowess in Haṭhayoga. They roam about on earth having transcended Time by the powers they acquired by mastering Hathayoga.

There are many Hatha Yoga masters. Just to hear their names is like getting their blessings. Above are some of the Hatha Yoga masters who attained the siddhis. They not only acquired powers, but more importantly, they were able to transcend time and space and to wander on all fourteen planes because they were able to take their prana into the Sushumna. Sometimes they come to the physical plane to help humanity, if you are ready for them. They could even keep their physical body alive if they wanted to by bringing the prana into the Sushumna. One can stop the decay of the physical person by stopping the Ida and Pingala and activating the Sushumna. Such a person, one whose energy moves through the Sushumna, is called a siddha. For him there is no day or night, no birth or death.

The Buddha referred to above is not the Buddha most of you know about. He is one of the Hatha Yoga masters.

अशेषतापतप्तानां समाश्रयमठो हठः ।
अशेषयोगयुक्तानामाधारकमठो हठः ॥ १० ॥

(10) Haṭhayoga is the refuge for all those scorched by the various types of pain. Haṭhayoga gives support to all those engaged in the constant practice of Yoga (as the tortoise in mythology) supports the whole of the planet earth.

हठविद्या परं गोप्या योगिना सिद्धिमिच्छता ।
भवेद्वीर्यवती गुप्ता निर्वीर्या तु प्रकाशिता ॥ ११ ॥

(11) Haṭhayoga-vidyā is to be greatly protected (kept hidden) by the yogī who desires perfection. (Only) when (thus) protected, is it effective (in generating siddhis); when not kept secret (hidden), it becomes ineffective.

This is a warning to keep the knowledge secret. Do not reveal it to just anybody. It is a vidya - a knowledge - something not meant for everybody unless they are ready. When the student comes to the teacher, the teacher judges whether he is ready. Moreover, this is not something for idle broadcasting. It is just for yourself. Your practice should not be revealed to anybody else as they will not understand. It is not for a public demonstration.

सुराज्ये धार्मिके देशे सुभिक्षे निरुपद्रवे ।
धनुःप्रमाणपर्यन्तं शिलाग्निजलवर्जिते ।
एकान्ते मठिकामध्ये स्थातव्यं हठयोगिना ॥ १२ ॥

(12) A Haṭhayoga practitioner should stay alone in a small place in a country (ruled) by a good (dhārmic) king, which is prosperous and which is free of troubles. The spot where Haṭhayoga is practiced should be free from stones, fire and water to the extent of the length of a bow.

The country should be one where the people are not gluttons, bandits or thugs. It must have a peaceful environment, one without terrorists, robbers or thieves. In a big city it is often dangerous to walk, but a country place is usually more suitable. "A country ruled over by a virtuous king" is one where the king is practicing dharma. Many countries are ruled over by dictators, and so they are places where it is legally forbidden to practice such things. I don't want to name them, but in certain countries you might be arrested for these practices. We must have full freedom to follow our practice without fear of disturbance.

You must also be situated in a place where food is available. You can't meditate or practice Hatha Yoga without sattvic foods such as lots of vegetables, fruit and milk.

"Free from rocks, water and fire": these are just very sensible instructions. The extent of a bow's length (how far an arrow can shoot) is maybe fifteen or twenty yards. Don't put your tent or other dwelling within twenty yards of a slope subject to falling rocks. Don't put your dwelling in an area subject to forest fires, earthquakes, or volcanoes. Don't put your tent near a swamp which will bring you the disturbances of mosquitoes and other pests. These are all sanitary considerations, not to be passed over lightly by anyone who wants to pursue this arduous course of Yoga.

अल्पद्वारमरन्ध्रगर्तविवरं नात्युच्चनीचायतं
सम्यग्गोमयसान्द्रलिप्तममलं निःशेषजन्तूज्झितम् ।

बाह्ये मण्डपवेदिकूपरुचिरं प्राकारसंवेष्टितं
प्रोक्तं योगमठस्य लक्षणमिदं सिद्धैर्हठाभ्यासिभिः ॥ १३ ॥

(13) The qualities of a yoga-maṭha (place where yoga is practiced) has been mentioned by the perfected ones practicing Haṭhayoga as follows: it should have a small entrance without windows, levelled and without holes; it should not be too high, too low or too deep; it should be clean (without dirt) smeared well with cow dung, free of all insects. Outside it should have a pleasant hall with a raised seat (and) a well; all this, in turn, should be surrounded by an outer wall.

एवंविधे मठे स्थित्वा सर्वचिन्ताविवर्जितः ।
गुरूपदिष्टमार्गेण योगवेम समभ्यसेत् ॥ १४ ॥

(14) Living in such a pleasant residence, devoid of any cares (thought) he should practice yoga in accordance with the teachings of his guru (or as taught by his guru).

It is not that the Yoga teacher is a baby-sitter, constantly watching. He is guiding you. You should begin pranayama only with the guidance of a guru. Otherwise you may not know the proper use of the diaphragm.

Merely studying all the books is not going to bring the desired result; you must practice. Many people read the **Bhagavad Gita** or **Ramayana** and they don't practice. Others read the **Bible** and then afterwards go and smoke. Such a course of action won't take you anywhere. Practice is important.

The siddhis are obtained from Lord Siva only when you are not planning to use those powers. At that time they come to you automatically. The siddhis or knowledge are given only to one who has devotion to the higher Self, not to the ego or to the body. Devotion to the guru is necessary also because God and guru are one. As God will not come directly to help, He has to manifest through your teacher. According to the nature of the teacher, the disciple relationship takes place. Some gurus you may have for only one day. Gurudev Sivananda's teacher had to stay for only one hour because Sivananda had already practiced in past lives. He became a great master after just a little further practice. Then, years later, when he touched me, all my past knowledge came, and he made me a Hatha Yoga professor. Master did not sit with me and teach all these things. I had been practicing from his Sadhana Tattva before that, but his presence was needed to bring back those past memories.

A teacher is needed to awaken this knowledge from samskaras (subtle impressions) of past lives. You are not just born ignorant or blind. The teacher opens samskaras either by touch, smell, teaching, etc. In ancient times this was the most usual way for the teacher to teach.

The teacher himself must have also gone through this training and disciplined his life so that he can apply that regimen to you. He must know how much he can give you because he sees your evolution. He must prescribe just like a doctor: perhaps a certain amount of japa to help reduce an overly rajasic nature, etc.

अत्याहार: प्रयासश्च प्रजल्पो नियमग्रह:।
जनसङ्गश्च लौल्यं च षड्भिर्योगो विनश्यति ॥ १५ ॥

(15) Yoga is destroyed through the following six (causes): over eating, too much fatigue, too mush talk, following unsuitable observances (niyama), keeping company with (unsuitable) people, and being fickle minded.

These are warnings. Certain things will not bring you success; they will not take you to the goal. Hard physical labor is one. When you are practicing intense asanas and pranayama, you cannot cut wood for ten hours. Just reduce it. A cold bath may be good at certain times, but not during intense pranayama. It will shatter your nerves. At such times only a warm bath is allowed. Also, you should not sit near a fire. Just as you cannot overload yourself with food during this intense sadhana, you may not fast for more than three to four hours at a time as this will weaken the body. You should have a moderate, balanced limited diet. Do not go to extremes. Also, do not eat before going to bed at night, because then in the early morning you will not be able to perform paranayama properly.

उत्साहात्साहसाद्धैर्यात्तत्त्वज्ञानाच्च निश्चयात् ।

जनसङ्गपरित्यागात् षड्भिर्योगः प्रसिध्यति ॥ १६ ॥

(16) Yoga flourishes with the following six (causes): enthusiasm, firm resolve, courage, knowledge of truth, determination, and giving up (abandoning) company of (unsuitable) people.

"True knowledge" is the knowledge that you are the Self (not the body), at least theoretically.

[To do no harm, to speak the truth, to refrain from taking what belongs to another, to preserve continence, to practice forbearance and fortitude, to be merciful to all, to be straightforward, to be moderate in diet, and to purify oneself - these constitute Yama.]

"Straightforwardly" means that in thought, word, and deed you practice the truth. Preserving continence (full brahmacharya) is especially important when you are practicing the intensive sadhana described in this book. Then you will be successful. It will be explained more a little later on. "Merciful" refers to ahimsa (non-violence).

[Tapas (austerities), cheerfulness, belief in God [astikya], charity, worship of the deity, hearing the exposition of Vedantic doctrines, shame, sound mind, japa (repeating prayers), and vratas (observance of vows) - these constitute niyama, the experts in Yoga say.]

हठस्य   प्रथमाङ्गत्वादासनं पूर्वमुच्यते।
कुर्यात्तदासनं स्थैर्यमारोग्यं चाङ्गलाघवम्॥ १७॥

*(17) Since they form the first stage of Haṭhayoga,
āsanas (postures) are mentioned to begin with.
Āsanas make one's body and mind steady, keep one
healthy and light of limb.*

By now you understand that asanas are not all of Hatha Yoga; they
are only the first stage.

वशिष्ठाद्यैश्च मुनिभिर्मत्स्येन्द्राद्यैश्च योगिभि:।
अङ्गीकृतान्यासनानि कथ्यन्ते कानिचिन्मया॥ १८॥

*(18) I shall (now) mention some āsanas which were
recognized by sages (munis) like Vasiṣṭha and others
and also by yogīs like Matsyendra and others.*

जानूर्वोरन्तरे   सम्यक्कृत्वा पादतले उभे।
ऋजुकाय: समासीन: स्वस्तिकं तत्प्रचक्षते॥ १९॥

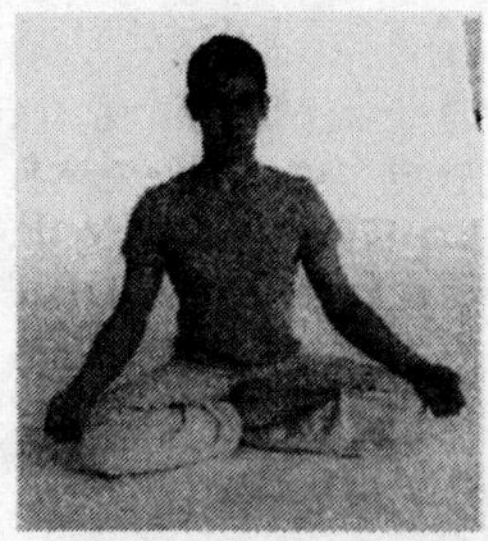

*(19) Keeping both the insteps of the feet
firmly between the thighs and the calves
of the legs, one should sit with body
straight on a level place. That is known
as Svastika (āsana).*

This is one of the meditative postures. Bend the right leg and bring
the foot in. Do the same with the left, placing it above the right leg.
Then place the toes of the left foot between the right calf and thigh.

सव्ये दक्षिणगुल्फं तु पृष्ठपार्श्वे नियोज्येत्।
दक्षिणेऽपि तथा सव्यं गोमुखं गोमुखाकृति॥ २०॥

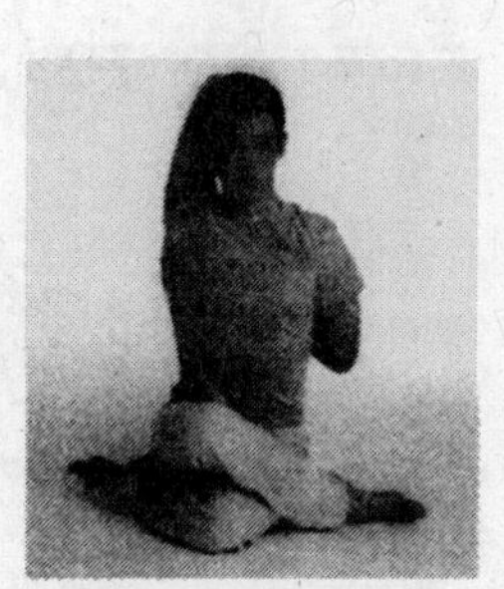

(20) Place the right ankle next to the left buttock and the left ankle next to the right buttock. This is called Gomukhāsana as it resembles the face of a cow.

एकं पादं तथैकस्मिन्विन्यसेदूरुणि स्थितम्।
इतरस्मिँस्तथा चोरुं वीरासनमितीरितम्॥ २१॥

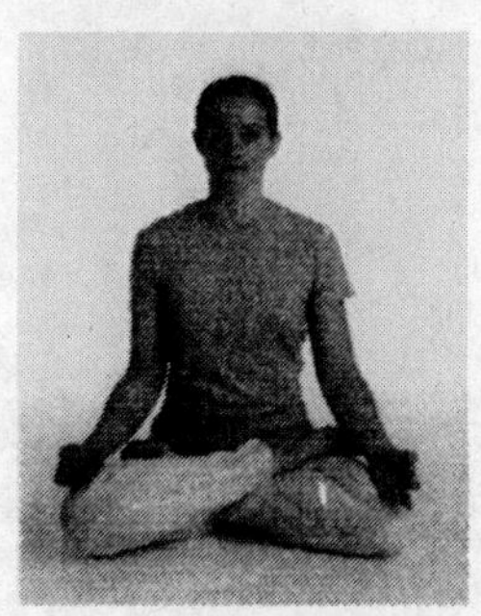

(21) Place the right foot on the other (left) thigh and the other (left) foot on the right thigh. This is Vīrāsana.

So it becomes the Lotus pose.

गुदं निरुध्यच गुल्फाभ्यां व्युत्क्रमेण समाहितः।
कूर्मासनं भवेदेतदिति योगविदो विदुः॥ २२॥

(22) Press the anus firmly with the soles crossed and sit very carefully. Yogīs call this the Kūrmāsana. (This resembles the tortoise)

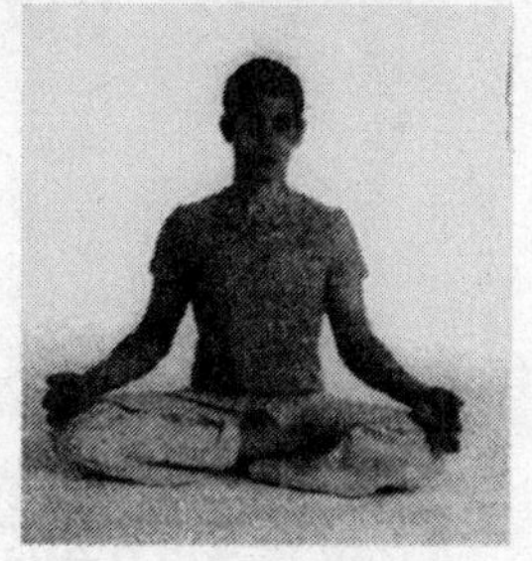

We call it Siddhasana. The above are the basic sitting poses.

पद्मासनं तु संस्थाप्य जानूर्वोरन्तरे करौ।
निवेश्य भूमौ संस्थाप्य व्योमस्थं कुक्कुटासनम्॥ २३॥

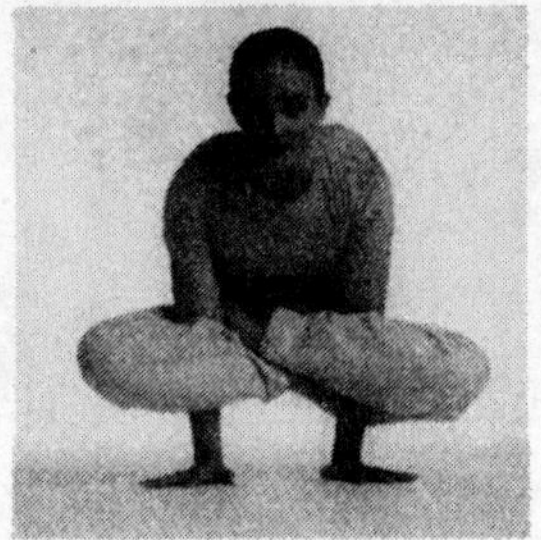

(23) After getting into the Padmāsana insert the hands between the thighs and calves. Plant the hands on the ground firmly and raise the body up. This is Kukkuṭāsana. (The chicken).

कुक्कुटासनबन्धस्थो दोर्भ्यां सम्बध्य कन्धराम्।
भवेत्कूर्मवदुत्तान एतदुत्तानकूर्मकम्॥ २४॥

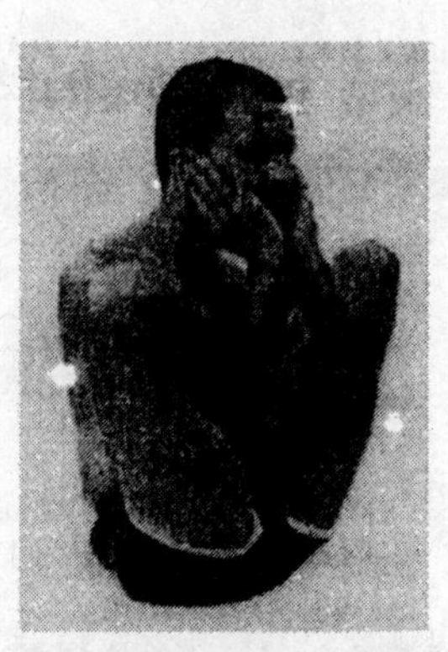

(24) Assuming Kukkuṭāsana, wind your arms around your neck and remain raised like a tortoise to the posture called Uttāna Kūrmāsana.

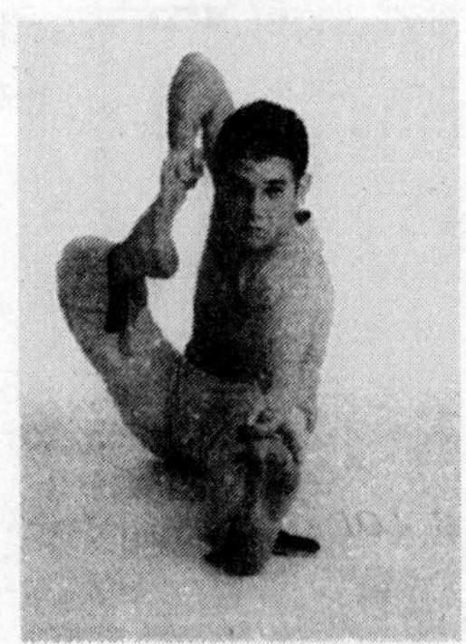

पादाङ्गुष्ठौ तु पाणिभ्यां गृहीत्वा श्रवणावधि।
धनुराकर्षणं　　　कुर्याद्धनुरासनमुच्यते॥ २५॥

(25) Taking hold of both the toes with your hands, keep one arm extended and draw the other towards your ear as you would do with the string of a bow. This is termed Dhanurāsana.

वामोरुमूलार्पितदक्षपादं　　　जानोर्बहिर्वेष्टितवामपादम्।
प्रगृह्य तिष्ठेत् परिवर्तिताङ्गः श्रीमत्स्यनाथोदितमासनं स्यात्॥ २६॥

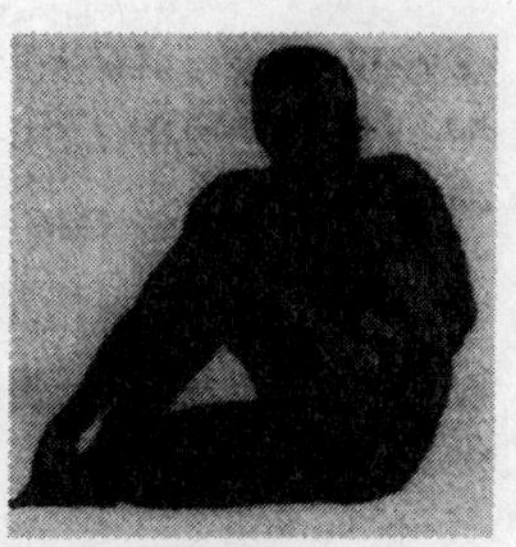

(26) Place the right foot at the root of the base of the left thigh and the left foot outside the right knee. Take hold of the right foot by the left hand and the left foot by the right hand and then turn your head towards the left completely. This is Matsyendrāsana.

मत्स्येन्द्रपीठं जठरप्रदीप्तिं प्रचण्डरुङ्‌मण्डलखण्डनास्त्रम् ।
अभ्यारात: कुण्डलिनीप्रबोधं चन्द्रस्थिरित्वं च ददाति पुंसाम् ॥ २७ ॥

(27) Matsyendrāsana is the weapon that destroys many terrible diseases and inflames the fire in the stomach (jaṭharāgni); it accomplishes the raising of Kuṇḍalinī and makes the moon steady when practiced regularly.

प्रसार्य पादौ भुवि दण्डरूपौ दोर्भ्यां पदाग्रद्वितयं गृहीत्वा ।
जानूपरिन्यस्तललाटदेशो   वसेदिदं पश्चिमतानमाहु: ॥ २८ ॥

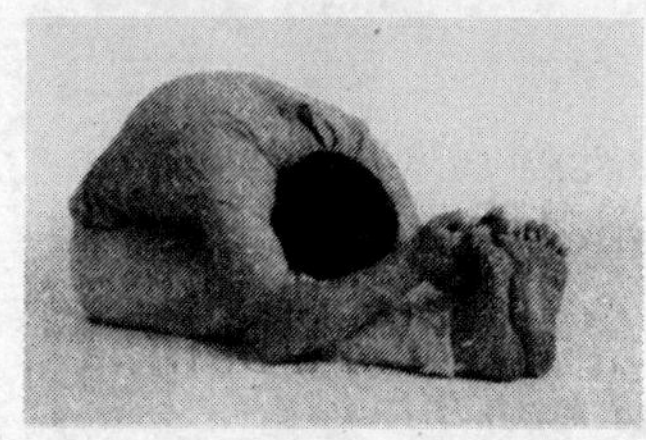

(28) Stretch out both the legs, and having taken hold of the toes of the feet with the hands, place your forehead upon your knees. This is Paścimatānāsana (or Paścimotthānāsana).

इति पश्चिमतानमासनाग्र्यं पवनं पश्चिमवाहिनं करोति ।
उदयं जठरानलस्य कुर्यादुदरे कार्श्यमरोगतां च पुंसाम् ॥ २९ ॥

(29) This important Paścimatānāsana makes the breath flow in the opposite direction (of suṣumnā). It causes the rise of the fire in the stomach; it causes leanness of the loins (stomach) and removes all diseases afflicting humans.

धरामवष्टभ्य   करद्वयेन   तत्कूर्परस्थापितनाभिपार्श्व: ।
उच्चासनो दण्डवदुत्थित: स्यान्मायूरमेतत्प्रवदन्ति पीठम् ॥ ३० ॥

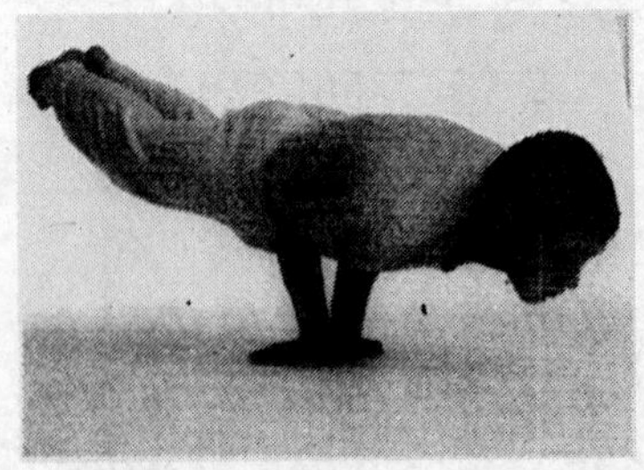

(30) Plant your hands firmly on the ground and support your body upon your elbows, pressing against the side of your loins. Raise your feet in the air stiff and straight and on a level with the head. This is Mayūrāsana.

हरति सकलरोगानाशुगुल्मोदरादी-
        नभिभवति च दोषानासनं श्रीमयूरम् ।
बहु कदशनभुक्तं भस्म कुर्यादशेषं
        जनयति जठराग्निं जारयेत्कालकूटम् ॥ ३१ ॥

(31) Mayūrāsana cures all diseases of the stomach, hands and spleen. It digests completely food taken in excess, it activates the interior fire (fire in the stomach) and even digests food which is (as destructive as) Halāhala (poison).

उत्तानं शववद्भूमौ शयनं तच्छवासनम् ।
शवासनं श्रान्तिहरं चित्तविश्रान्तिकारकम् ॥ ३२ ॥

*(32) Lying flat on the ground on the back like a
corpse is Śavāsana. This āsana removes fatigue
(caused by the āsanas) and induces mental peace.*

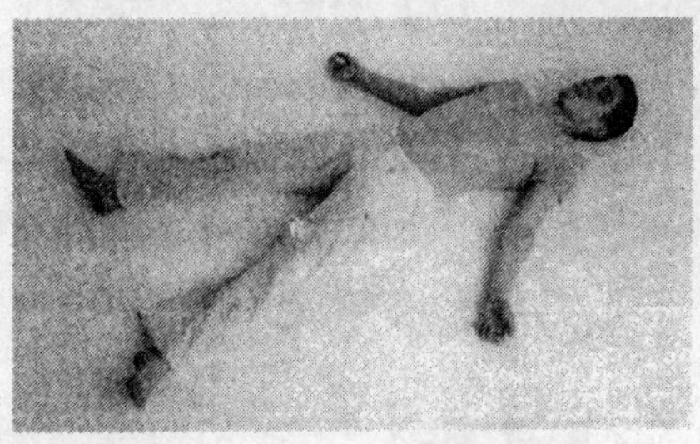

चतुरशीत्यासनानि शिवेन कथितानि च।
तेभ्यश्चतुष्कमादाय सारभूतं ब्रवीम्यहम्॥ ३३॥

*(33) Lord Śiva has described 84 āsanas.
I shall explain four of the most important of those.*

सिद्धं   पद्मं तथा सिंहं भद्रं चेति चतुष्टयम्।
श्रेष्ठं तत्रापि च सुखे तिष्ठेत् सिद्धासने सदा॥ ३४॥

*(34) They are: Siddha, Padma, Siṃha, and Bhadra.
Of these the most comfortable and the most excellent
is Siddhāsana.*

योनिस्थानकमङ्घ्रिमूलघटितं कृत्वा दृढं विन्यसे-
        न्मेढ्रेपादमथैकमेव हृदये कृत्वा हनुं सुस्थिरम्।
स्थाणुः संयमितेन्द्रियोऽचलदृशा पश्येद् भ्रुवोरन्तरं
        ह्येतन्मोक्षकपाटभेदजनकं सिद्धासनं प्रोच्यते॥ ३५॥

*(35) Press firmly the perineal space with the heel and
place the other heel above the pubic bones. Fix your*

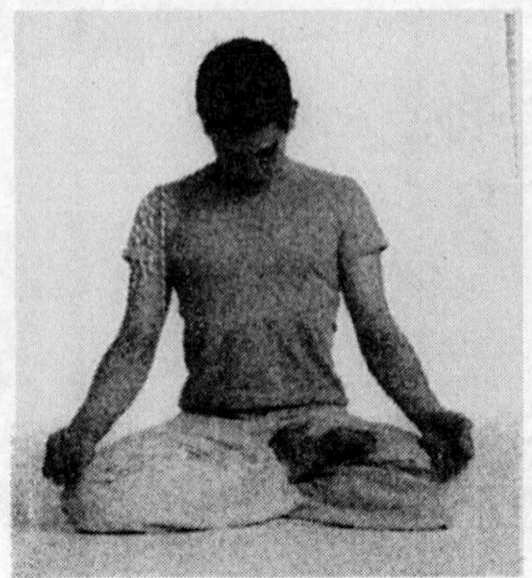

chin tightly upon your chest. Remain with back straight up with your organs under control and look fixedly at the spot between the eyebrows. This is called Siddhāsana. This āsana removes every obstacle from the path to mokṣa (liberation).

मेढ्रादुपरि विन्यस्य सव्यं गुल्फं तथोपरि।
गुल्फान्तरं च निक्षिप्य सिद्धासनमिदं भवेत्॥ ३६॥

(36) Place the right heel above the pubic bone and the left heel above the right heel. This is also called Siddhāsana.

The one now described is preferred by other yogis.

एतत् सिद्धासनं प्राहुरन्ये वज्रासनं विदुः।
मुक्तासनं वदन्त्येके प्राहुर्गुप्तासनं परे॥ ३७॥

(37) This is called Siddhāsana; others know it as Vajrāsana. It is also called Muktāsana or Guptāsana.

यमेष्विव मिताहारमहिंसां नियमेष्विव।
मुख्यं सर्वासनेष्वेकं सिद्धाः सिद्धासनं विदुः॥ ३८॥

(38) The siddhas say that as among niyamas the most important is ahiṃsā, and among yamas a moderate diet, so is Siddhāsana among āsanas.

चतुरशीतिपीठेषु सिद्धमेव सदाभ्यसेत्।
द्वासप्ततिसहस्राणां नाडीनां मलशोधनम्॥ ३९॥

(39) Of the 84 āsanas, one should always practice Siddhāsana. It purifies the 72,000 nādīs.

आत्माध्यायी मिताहारी यावद्द्वादशवत्सरम्।
सदा सिद्धासनाभ्यासाद्योगी निष्पत्तिमाप्नुयात्॥ ४०॥

(40) If the yogī regularly sits in Siddhāsana for twelve years, stays with a moderate diet while contemplating on his Ātman constantly, he will surely attain perfection in Yoga.

किमन्यैर्बहुभिः पीठैः सिद्धे सिद्धासने सति।
प्राणानिले सावधाने बद्धे केवलकुम्भके॥ ४१॥

उत्पद्यते निरायासात्स्वयमेवोन्मनी कला।
तथैकस्मिन्नेव दृढे सिद्धे सिद्धासने सति।
बन्धत्रयमनायासात्स्वयमेवोपजायते   ॥ ४२॥

(41) When Siddhāsana is mastered and the breath carefully restrained by the practice of Kevala Kumbhaka, then arises without any effort the avasthā known as Unmanī.

(42) When Siddhāsana is mastered, the three bandhas follow naturally without effort.

नासनं सिद्धसदृशं न कुम्भ: केवलोपम: ।
न खेचरी समा मुद्रा न नादसदृशो लय: ॥ ४३ ॥

(43) There is no āsana like Siddhāsana, no kumbhaka like the Kevala, no mudrā like the Khecarī, and no laya (absorption of the mind) like the Nāda.

वामोरूपरि   दक्षिणं च चरणं संस्थाप्य वामं तथा ।
दक्षोरूपरि पश्चिमेन विधिना धृत्वा कराभ्यां दृढम् ।
अङ्गुष्ठौ हृदये निधाय चिबुकं नासाग्रमालोकये-
देतद्व्याधिविनाशकारि यमिनां पद्मासनं प्रोच्यते ॥ ४४ ॥

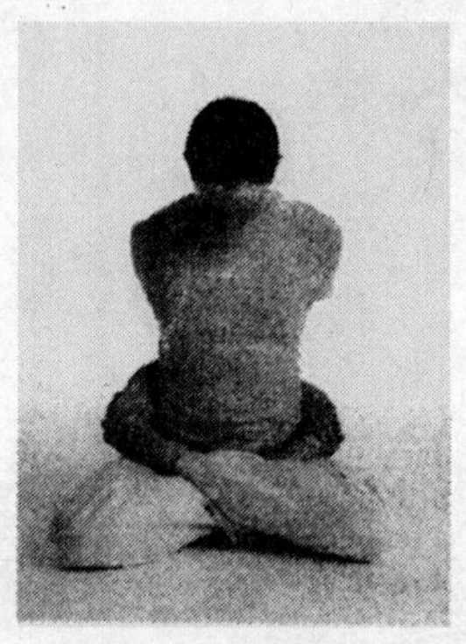

(44) Place the right heel at the root of the left thigh and the left heel at the root of the right. Cross the hands behind the back and take hold of the toes (the right toe with the right hand and the left toe with the left). Place the chin firmly on the chest and look fixedly at the tip of the nose. This is called Padmāsana; this destroys all diseases.

उत्तानौ चरणौ कृत्वा ऊरुसंस्थौ प्रयत्नत: ।
ऊरुमध्ये तथोत्तानौ पाणी कृत्वा ततो दृशौ ॥ ४५ ॥

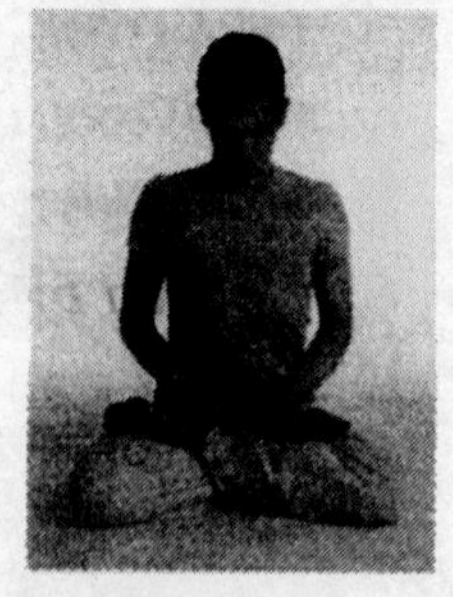

नासाग्रे विन्यसेद्राजदन्तमूले तु जिह्वया ।
उत्तम्भ्य चिबुकं वक्षस्युत्थाप्य पवनं शनै: ॥ ४६ ॥

(45 and 46) An alternate version of Padmāsana: Place the feet firmly (soles up) on the opposite thighs

and place the hands (palms up) one upon another in between the thighs. Direct your eyes to the top of the nose and place the tip of the tongue at the root of the front teeth. Place the chin on the chest and slowly raise upwards the prāṇa.

इदं पद्मासनं प्रोक्तं सर्वव्याधिविनाशनम्।
दुर्लभं येन केनापि धीमता लभ्यते भुवि॥ ४७॥

(47) This is Padmāsana that destroys all diseases. It cannot be attained by ordinary mortals. Only some intelligent (wise, courageous) persons attain it.

कृत्वा सम्पुटितौ करौ दृढतरं बद्ध्वा तु पद्मासनं
        गाढं वक्षसि सन्निधाय चिबुकं ध्यायँश्च तच्चेतसि।
वारं वारमपानमूर्ध्वमनिलं प्रोत्सारयन्पूरितं
        न्यञ्चन्प्राणमुपैति बोधमतुलं शक्ति प्रभावान्नरः॥ ४८॥

(48) Assuming Padmāsana and having placed the palms one upon another, fix the chin firmly upon the chest and practice meditation, frequently contract the anus and raise the apāna upwards. By a similar contraction of the throat, force the prāṇa downwards. By this the yogī obtains unequalled knowledge through the favor of (Kuṇḍalinī) Śakti (which is roused by this process).

पद्मासने स्थितो योगी नाडीद्वारेण पूरितम्।
मारुतं धारयेद्यस्तु स मुक्तो नात्र संशयः॥ ४९॥

(49) The Yogī, sitting in the Padmāsana by restraining the breath drawn in through the nāḍīs, becomes liberated. This is beyond doubt.

गुल्फौ च वृषणस्याधः सीवन्याः पार्श्वयोः क्षिपेत् ।
दक्षिणे सव्यगुल्फं तु दक्षगुल्फं तु सव्यके ॥५०॥

हस्तौ तु जान्वोः संस्थाप्य स्वाङ्गुलीः संप्रसार्य च ।
व्यात्तवक्त्रो निरीक्षेत नासाग्रं सुसमाहितः ॥५१॥

सिंहासनं भवेदेतत्पूजितं योगिपुङ्गवैः ।
बन्धत्रितयसन्धानं कुरुते चासनोत्तमम् ॥५२॥

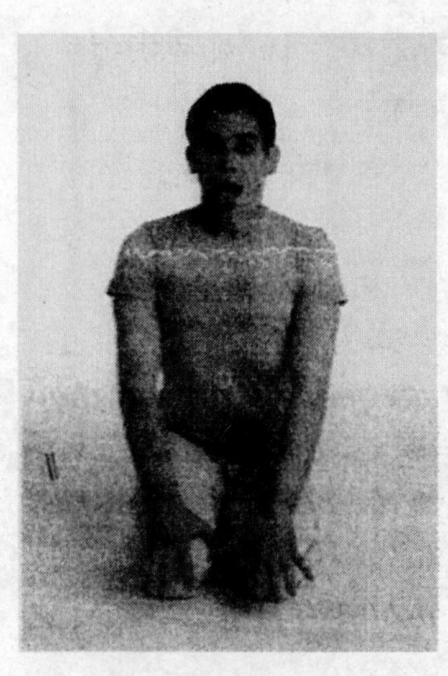

(50-52) Now the Siṃhāsana is described: Place the ankles at the perineum - right ankle upon the left side of it, and the left ankle upon the right. Place the palms upon the knees, extend the fingers and direct the eyes to the tip of the nose with opened mouth and a concentrated mind. This is the Siṃhāsana held in great esteem by the highest yogīs. This most excellent āsana facilitates the three bandhas.

गुल्फौ च वृषणस्याधः सीवन्याः पार्श्वयोः क्षिपेत् ।
सव्यगुल्फं तथा सव्ये दक्षगुल्फं तु दक्षिणे ॥५३॥

पार्श्वपादौ च पाणिभ्यां दृढं बद्ध्वा सुनिश्चलम् ।
भद्रासनं   भवेदेतत्सर्वव्याधिविनाशनम् ॥ ५४ ॥

गोरक्षासनमित्याहुरिदं वै सिद्धयोगिनः ।
एवमासनबन्धेषु योगीन्द्रो विगतश्रमः ॥ ५५ ॥

This is the main thing. After performing asanas, now you must purify the nadis, the nerves. That is what the second chapter instructs.

अभ्यसेन्नाडिकाशुद्धिं   मुद्रादिपवनक्रियाम् ।
आसनं कुम्भकं चित्रं मुद्राख्यं करणं तथा ॥ ५६ ॥

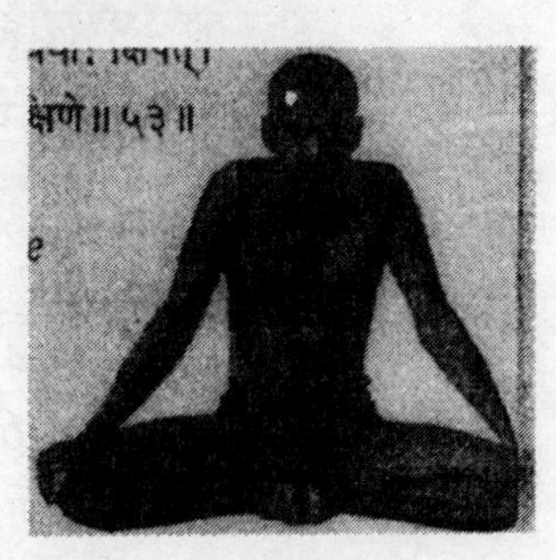

(53-56) Now the Bhadrāsana: Place the ankles upon the sides of the perineum; the right upon the right and the left on the left. Then hold firmly with your hands the feet which are on their side.
This āsana destroys all ills. This is also called Gorakṣāsana by Siddhas and Yogīs. The Yogī free from pain and fatigue in practising these āsanas relentlessly should (then) practise purification of the nāḍīs, mudrās, control of breath etc.

So after pranayama, we go into meditation. Here it takes the form of concentration on the inner sound. We will go into this later on.

अथ   नादानुसन्धानमभ्यासानुक्रमो   हठे ।
ब्रह्मचारी   मिताहारी   त्यागी   योगपरायणः ।
अब्दादूर्ध्वं भवेत् सिद्धो नात्र कार्या विचारणा ॥ ५७ ॥

*Then (in the course of Haṭhayoga) the āsanas,
prāṇāyāma, kumbhakas, mudrās etc., then
concentration upon the nāda (the anāhata sounds
which come from the Anāhata Cakra or the cardiac
plexus) comes next.*

*(57) The brahmacārī observing a moderate diet, being
devoted to Yoga and having a detached temperament
becomes a siddha after a year. There need be no doubt
about this.*

For this you must practice all these things properly.

सुस्निग्धमधुराहारश्चचतुर्थांशविवर्जितः ।
भुज्यते शिवसम्प्रीत्यै मिताहारः स उच्यते ॥ ५८ ॥

*(58) For the sake of pleasing Lord Śiva,
one eats pleasant and sweet food moderately
leaving one fourth of the stomach free.*

कट्वम्लतीक्ष्णलवणोष्णहरीतशाकसौवीरतैलतिलसर्षपमद्यमत्स्यान् ।
आजादिमांसदधितक्रकुलत्थकोलपिण्याकहिङ्गुलशुनाद्यमपथ्यमाहुः ॥ ५९ ॥

*(59) The following food items are prohibited for a
Yogī: food that is sharp, sour, pungent and hot, viz.,
myrobalan, betel nut and betel leaves, sour gruel,
sesame or mustard oil, liquors, fish, flesh of animals
like goat etc., curds, buttermilk, fruit of the jujube, oil
cakes, asafoetida and garlic.*

These things should be avoided during a course of intense
pranayama such as this one.

भोजनमहितं विद्यात् पुनरस्योष्णीकृतं रूक्षम्।
अतिलवणमम्लयुक्तं कदशनशाकोत्कटं वर्ज्यम्॥ ६०॥

(60) The following unhealthy food items should be avoided: stale and reheated, very dry and very sour food; also, food that is very difficult to digest, and that has too many vegetables.

Food that has once been cooked should not be reheated as that will drive out all its energy. This rule originated because there was no refrigeration in India, and people would leave food from one meal to the next and then reheat it – something very bad. Indigestible.

वह्निस्त्रीपथिसेवानामादौ वर्जनमाचरेत्॥ ६१॥
तथाहि गोरक्षवचनम्–
''वर्जयेद्दुर्जनप्रान्तं वह्निस्त्रीपथिसेवनम्।
प्रातःस्नानोपवासादि कायक्लेशविधिं तथा।''

(61) This is what Gorakṣa says: The Yogī should avoid basking by the fire, company of women, long journeys, early morning baths, fasting and hard physical work.

Basking near a fire will cause you to inhale carbon dioxide.

गांधूमशालियवषष्टिकशोभनान्नं क्षीराज्यखण्डनवनीतसितामधूनि।
शुण्ठीपटोलकफलादिकपञ्चशाकं मुद्रादिदिव्यमुदकं च यमीन्द्रपथ्यम्॥ ६२॥

(62) The following is permitted for a Yogī: Wheat, rice, barley, milk, ghee, sugar candy, butter, honey, dry ginger, cucumber, the five potherbs, green gram and good clean water.

Ghee is clarified butter. Sugar candy is a crystallized form of sugar. Cucumber is one of the best things you can take. Your Western spinach is one of the five potherbs mentioned.

पुष्टं सुमधुरं स्निग्धं गव्यं धातुप्रपोषणम् ।
मनोऽभिलषितं योग्यं योगी भोजनमाचरेत् ॥ ६३ ॥

(63) Food that is sweet and mixed with milk is nourishing for the Yogī; this would be pleasant and nutritive at the same time.

This is very important. We give it to our sadhana intensive students in the early morning to help their pranayama. It is very nourshing and not at all heavy.

युवा वृद्धोऽतिवृद्धो वा व्याधितो दुर्बलोऽपि वा ।
अभ्यासात्सिद्धिमाप्नोति   सर्वयोगेष्वतन्द्रितः ॥ ६४ ॥

(64) Any person, who giving up laziness, practices assiduously all the yogāsanas will attain perfection be he young, old or even very old, sickly and weak.

Anyone who is able to get control of the prana, be he young, old, or even every sickly and weak, can get success.

क्रियायुक्तस्य सिद्धिः स्यादक्रियस्य कथं भवेत् ।
न   शास्त्रपाठमात्रेण   योगसिद्धिः   प्रजायते ॥ ६५ ॥

(65) Siddhis are obtained only with unstinted work at Yogic kriyās; Yogic siddhis are not achieved by merely reading the texts. How can one who does not do them attain perfection?

न वेषधारणं सिद्धेः कारणं न च तत्कथा।
क्रियैव कारणं सिद्धेः सत्यमेतन्न संशय॥ ६६ ॥

*(66) By just putting on the Yogic attire (or props),
one does not become a siddha. Nor does he get it by
merely talking about it. Practice of yoga makes a
perfect yogī. This is without doubt.*

Merely wearing an orange robe and growing a beard will not do
it; you are still the same person underneath.

*or by talking about them, but untiring practice is the
secret of success. There is not doubt about this.*

पीठानि कुम्भकाश्चित्रा दिव्यानि करणानि च।
सर्वाण्यपि हठाभ्यासे राजयोगफलावधि ॥ ६७ ॥

इति श्री सहजानन्दसन्तानचिन्तामणिस्वात्मारामयोगीन्द्रविरचितायां
हठयोगप्रदीपिकायां आसनविधिकथनं नाम प्रथमोपदेशः ॥

*(67) Āsanas, kumbhakas and mudrās of Hathayoga
should be practiced meticulously till one attains
Rājayoga.*

Thus ends the first chapter entitled Āsanavidhikathanam of *Hatha
Yoga Pradīpīkā* authored by Svātmārāma Yogīndra the brilliant-
jewel of the son of Sahajānanda.

These should be practiced until the mind becomes very steady and
the prana goes into the Sushumna. Until then you must practice.
Just practice. Don't keep looking for a result; from practice and more
practice, eventually it will come. If you lift weights every day, little
by little your muscles will develop. It is the same here.

हठयोगप्रदीपिका

Hatha Yoga Pradīpīkā

CHAPTER TWO

अथासने दृढे योगी वशी हितमिताशनः ।
गुरूपदिष्टमार्गेण प्राणायामान् समभ्यसेत् ॥ १ ॥

(1) After gaining through proficiency in all the postures, exercising control over the senses, consuming moderate diet. the aspirant (yogī) should follow the instructions of his guru in the breathing exercises known as prāṇāyāma.

अथासने दृढे योगी वशी हितमिताशन: ।
गुरुपदिष्टमार्गेण प्राणायामान् समभ्यसेत् ॥ १ ॥

(1) After gaining through proficiency in all the postures, exercising control over the senses, consuming moderate diet, the aspirant (yogī) should follow the instructions of his guru in the breathing exercises known as prāṇāyāma.

चले वाते चलं चित्तं निश्चले निश्चलं भवेत् ।
योगीस्थाणुत्वमाप्नोति   ततो वायुं निरोधयेत् ॥ २ ॥

(2) When the breathing is unsteady, the mind is also unsteady. But when the breath is steady, the mind attains steadiness. Then, it will give a long and healthy life. Therefore, the yogī should practice prāṇāyāma.

How can the breath wander? We can understand this verse only when we realize that it is not the physical breath that is meant here, it is the prana. This confusion is due to the problems of translation. The original Sanskrit, "Prana Vayu," is here translated as breath because in English there is no word for prana. Sometimes it is translated as air, other times as breath. Because of possibilities of confusion such as this, a guru is necessary.

Mind is like a tree and breath is like the wind. We can't see the wind, but when we see the motion of the tree, we know that the air is disturbed. It is the same with thought. When the prana is disturbed or unsteady, your mind is so disturbed that you cannot sit quietly in one place. In the extreme case of a madman, the prana is so very disturbed that it is not being channelled properly (neither afferent nor efferent currents are moving correctly, and the motor or sensory nerves are out of control). Then thought and body actions are completely out of control and one talks, moves and laughs completely inappropriately. This also happens to all of us in different degrees whenever our minds are not completely steady – when "breath wanders." The important thing to understand here is the prana and mind are interconnected.

The Pradipika says that "One should restrain the breath," but you all know that if you do that literally you won't live long. Again, we see that we must translate breath as prana. When this prana is regulated so that it becomes rhythmic, then breath also becomes rhythmic. We can watch the physical breath to learn how the prana moves. From watching the leaves on the tree, we know whether the wind is from the north or from the south, whether its speed is eight knots or whether it is stormy. Similarly, by watching the physical breath, we can tell a person's mental condition. This is one of the principles upon which lie detector machines are based.

When you do pranayama you are regulating the impulse coming to the diaphragm in a proportional way (1:4:2). Impulses are always going from the brain to the rest of the body, as for example when I move my arm. You cannot see the impulse but you can see the motion. The muscle is controlled by the mind which sends the impulses through the nervous system to the muscles. It all depends upon thought as it is thought which controls the impulses.

By using the physical breath you are regulating the impulse of prana (and of apana as well). Then, with the contraction of Mula bandha you are trying to stop the impulse from going to the sexual and lower organs; you are bringing the energy up. You shut off the prana not only by holding the breath, but also by touching the chin to the chest. By putting pressure on various nerves, you control the cardiovascular system: the heart rate and the respiratory rate. When you put pressure on the Muladhara chakra by pressing the anal sphincter muscle with the heel and by sitting over that area, you are putting pressure on the Kanda, the place where all the nerves are joined. This presses on the apana, forcing it up. The prana is forced down by the chin lock. In this way these two impulses are joined together. That is called Hatha Yoga, the union of "ha" and "tha." We need to apply physical pressure as well as to employ the mind and the breath. Breath, thought, and body are all employed; then with all three together, you get full control.

It is said that if you are very advanced in Raja Yoga, you don't have to go through this process. An advanced Raja yogi is one who can control his thought; once you do that, you control everything –

prana and the body. But such a person is very rare. An advanced Raja yogi has full control over the emotions: lust, anger, greed, hatred, jealousy, envy, fear. Most of us need to practice Hatha Yoga in order to get to Raja Yoga.

The yogi is said to "live long" because he regulates the impulse coming so that the breath slows. In proportion that breath slows, life is prolonged, because then energy is burned up more slowly. Catabolic and anabolic activity both go down, one is balanced, and so youth is maintained for a long time.

यावद्वायुः स्थितो देहे तावज्जीवनमुच्यते।
मरणं तस्य निष्क्रान्तिस्ततो वायुं निरोधयेत्॥ ३॥

(3) Till such time breath stays in the body,
one is said to be active; the moment breathing stops,
death ensues. So, one should practice prāṇāyāma.

Again, he is not talking about the physical breath, but about prana.

मलाकुलासु नाडीषु मारुतो नैव मध्यगः।
कथं स्यादुन्मनीभावः कार्यसिद्धिः कथं भवेत्॥ ४॥

(4) When the nāḍīs are full of impurities,
the breath does not enter the middle nāḍī,
(the suṣumnā nāḍī); then, how can one achieve
the goal of entering Unmanī-Avasthā?

Modern people who read such things may think that the author is making a ridiculous statement, that he knows nothing about physiology or anatomy. How can breath possibly go into the nadi when everybody knows that it goes only into the lungs! But if you again translate "breath" as prana, as I have explained, then you will understand such things properly.

What are the "impurities" mentioned above? When you eat the wrong food, when you drink or smoke, the nervous system is loaded with impurities, creating resistance. At that time, if you do pranayama, the prana will not go into the Sushumna. If the breath doesn't go into the Sushumna nadi, then there is "no attainment of the object." What is meant by that? The "object" is the union of "ha" and "tha," the union that will lead to stillness of the mind. When the mind is still, Raja yogis say that the seer sees Himself. He sees Himself as "I Am."

Unmani avasta is Hatha Yoga samadhi through control of the prana. In Raja Yoga this same state is called Asamprajnata Samadhi. In Jnana Yoga it is called Nirvikalpa Samadhi or Turiya. In Bhakti Yoga it is called Bhava Samadhi or self-surrender. All are the same state.

During Unmani avasta the breath stops and the mind becomes so still that you see the Self. Avastha refers to a state of the mind. In this state there are no more waves (vrittis) in the mind because the prana is no longer working through the Ida and Pingala. So long as the prana operates through these nadis, there will be physical breathing and life force, emotions and thoughts. Ordinarily we cannot stop this; it stops only when the prana goes in the Sushumna so that Ida and Pingla are dead. Then they are like a wire without any current.

शुद्धिमेति यदा सर्वं नाडीचक्रं महाकुलम् ।
तदैव   जायते योगी प्राणसङ्ग्रहणे क्षमः ॥ ५ ॥

(5) When all the nāḍīs, which are very impure,

become purified, only then can the yogī attain mastery

of prāṇāyāma.

"Successfully" means that the prana goes into the Sushumna. When the nadis are impure, prana will not go into the Sushumna, so we must begin by doing pranayama to purification; the rest comes automatically. Actually, most of the time we spend in purification.

प्राणायामं   ततः कुर्यान्नित्यं सात्त्विकया धिया ।
यथा सुषुम्नानाडीस्था मलाः शुद्धिं प्रयान्ति च ॥ ६ ॥

(6) With the mind in a sāttvic (tranquil) state,
prāṇāyāma should be practiced daily so that the
impurities present in suṣumnā nāḍī are removed and
the nāḍī becomes clear.

The "sattvic element" prevails when you want to reach your Self, or God, and are not performing pranayama for getting siddhis or powers. If these were your goal, then it would be the rajo-guna which would predominate. But this would be like the left hand trying to dominate the right hand, when actually there is only one Self. So if I want to show that I am bigger than you, that's not power, it's only illusion, ignorance. We should be performing this sadhana in order to reach the Self.

until the Sushumna nadi is freed from the impurities.

That may take one life, ten lives, ten million lives, or just ten seconds– that's possible too. How do you know that you have awakened this purification? The first sign is contentment. Do you know what is contentment? If you started this practice, hoping to gain a mink coat, by the time you are finished, you don't need or want a mink coat. You don't want anything. You got what you were really looking for: peace and self-contentment. When a person achieves this, he doesn't have to go to a bar or a discotheque or a concert. He is content to just look at a tree or to sit in a bare room. He is satisfied in whatever conditions he finds himself. If there's no electricity, that's okay. If there's no hot water, it's all right. But if tomorrow suddenly a beautiful dinner and wonderful dishes were brought, that would be okay too. That's called contentment.

When you are contented you are not looking for something, expecting happiness only if you have such and such a thing. For example, only if the weather is good, are you going to be happy. Only if Swami Vishnu teaches you everything are you going to be happy; only if your husband buys you a mink coat are you going to be happy; only if your wife cooks a delicious meal are you going to be happy.

In that way, will you ever find happiness? No, because when you are depending on someone else, things can always go wrong, and they do. You can't expect the sun to come out just because you are not happy without. But you can be happy within your Self. You can smile at the rain also. That's called contentment.

When the nadis are purified, your thoughts are no longer going from right brain to left brain, and left brain to right brain. There is balance, there are no more ups and downs. Usually our life swings like a pendulum: one day going this – happy and jumping and joyful, the next day going that way. Like a yo-yo, back and forth and back and forth. But Yoga is a balanced state of mind. Then hot and cold are the same, victory and defeat the same, censure and praise the same, gain and loss the same. That's called contentment.

When the prana goes in the Sushumna, the first sign is contentment. You can be alone in a cave as I was, or if you have to come and work with people, that's all right too. One day I was in a cave in the Himalayas and I was contented. The next day I was in a five star hotel in London. A five star hotel is all right too, but that hotel was just a temporary abode and not the source of my contentment. In the cave there was no hot or even cold water. I had to melt snow for water. Every day I had to be careful with firewood as it was very hard to find and extremely expensive to buy. But that was okay – that was the way God wanted it. And even though everybody had gone and I was alone, I was contented, knowing that I was an independent person and I could be happy by myself.

This comes naturally when purification has taken place and the Kundalini is slowly moving in an upward direction. In the downward direction it is a yo-yo. This is how you will know it. As an example, suppose after eating a full meal, suddenly you were brought more food, what would you do? You wouldn't care about it, because the desire for food is gone. It is the same with purification of the nadis. It comes automatically.

When peace and contentment come to you, it means that the Kundalini is awakened or the Shakti is opened. Then you radiate this peace. Your friends and your family will see something new in you – a peaceful and calm face. They will sense a new atmosphere. They will feel just like a cold person coming from outside and warming himself in front of a fireplace. If you feel this contentment, others will also feel it. But even if others don't feel it, you are not unhappy about it because everyone is not going to praise you. Some people are going to criticise you anyway. That's the way the world is – the world of duality. No one ever is always praised in this world by everybody. Can you tell me of just one person who was praised by everybody? Was Moses praised by everybody? Even after forty years, among his own people there were many who revolted against him. Did everyone praise Jesus? They crucified him even though he was talking about peace and love. Similarly, Krishna, Rama, Buddha and Socrates were criticized. Swami Sivananda was criticized by his disciples; someone even brought an axe against him.

Your happiness should not be depending on outside influences. It is not ego if you have confidence in your own Self. Confidence in the Self means that you are seeing that one Self in everything as all are one. Then you know that there's nothing to please. The moment you are really satisfied with your life, it means that your Kundalini has awakened and your Sushumna is purified.

बद्धपद्मासनो   योगी प्राणं चन्द्रेण पूरयेत्।
धारयित्वा यथाशक्ति भूयः सूर्येण रेचयेत् ॥ ७ ॥

(7) Seated in padmāsana, the yogī should draw in the prāṇa through the left nostril called the Moon (or the iḍā) and hold it as long as one can; the breath then should be exhaled through the right nostril called the sun (or the piṅgalā.)

प्राणं सूर्येण चाकृष्य पूरयेदुदरं   शनैः।
विधिवत्स्तम्भकं कृत्वा पुनश्चन्द्रेण रेचयेत् ॥ ८ ॥

(8) Again inhaling through the right nostril, he should fill the stomach with air slowly; then practicing kumbhakam (stoppage of breath) as given in the sacred texts, the breath should be released through the left nostril.

येन त्यजेत्तेन पीत्वा धारयेदतिरोधतः ।
रेचयेच्च ततोऽन्येन शनैरेव न वेगतः ॥ ९ ॥

(9) He should perform pūraka (inhalation) through the same nostril by which he performed recaka (exhalation), and having retained the breath to the utmost, he should exhale it slowly through the other nostril; release of breath should be done slowly and never in a fast manner.

प्राणं चेदिडया पिबेन्नियमितं भूयोऽन्यया रेचयेत् ।
पीत्वा पिङ्गलया समीरणमथो बद्ध्वा त्यजेद्वामया ।
सूर्याचन्द्रमसोरनेन विधिनाऽभ्यासं सदा तन्वतां
शुद्धा नाडिगणा भवन्ति यमिनां मासत्रयादूर्ध्वतः ॥ १० ॥

(10) If the prāṇa is drawn in by the left (iḍā), it is ordained that it should be exhaled by the other. Again, having taken the breath through the right pingalā, and having retained it as long as possible, it should be exhaled through the left. The yogī should continuously practice control of the breath of Sun and Moon (Sūrya and Chandra breaths) by this method. (Then) in the case of such self controlled yogīs, the entire nāḍīs become purified within three months.

This is Anuloma Viloma [Alternate Nostril Breathing]. In three months you can achieve a certain degree of purification. There will be satisfaction, peace and contentment. All this will come, provided you have this qualification: observance of yamas and niyamas. Merely practising left and right breathing alone is not sufficient.

What are the niyama? They are the following observances:

(1) Saucha – cleanliness, both internal and external: internal

cleaning through Neti and Dhauti, and a sattvic, pure vegetarian diet.

(2) Santosha – contentment (discussed before), where you are satisfied in whatever situation you are. Some person may be born in a big place and another may be born in a slum. What is the cause behind it? Karma. It is our own actions from the past which cause reaction. So you should be contented no matter what situation you are thrown into.

(3) Tapas – Penance (fasting, taking vows such as performing a certain number of asanas, pranayamas, or eating only a certain type of food). No foolish vows like standing in the cold water for ten hours and sitting in the hot sun near a burning fire. Some foolish people do these things, but that's torture and it's against Yoga. True yogis won't do that type of tapas. Torturing the body in the name of God is not allowed. Neither is surrounding the body with too much luxury. Follow the middle path: not too much luxury, not too much suffering.

(4) Swadyaya – study of the scriptures.

(5) Ishwarapranidana – surrender to the will of God or surrender of the ego.

These are the yamas, or restrictions:

(1) Satyam – telling the truth.

(2) Ahimsa – non-violence.

(3) Brahmacharya – celibacy.

(4) Asteya – non-covetousness.

(5) Aparigraha – non-receiving of presents.

Once the yamas and niyamas are established, then you perform pranayama. Only under this condition will you get the purification within three months. Anyone can practice pranayama, but if yama and niyama are not there, success will not come easily because mind will not be going in the right direction. But if those conditions are met, you can get the benefits even now; a tremendous inner awakening may come at any time.

प्रातर्मध्यन्दिने सायमर्धरात्रे च कुम्भकान् ।
शनैरशीतिपर्यन्तं चतुर्वारं समभ्यसेत् ॥ ११ ॥

(11) Kumbhakas should be performed four times daily, viz., early morning, midday, evening and midnight. Increase the rounds (gradually) to eighty.

This means that at these four times during the day one should practice this inhalation, retention, exhalation, until perspiration comes. As the proportions are increased, you will feel perspiration coming out.

until he increases the number to eighty.

That's forty rounds, one round containing two retentions. Forty rounds make eighty retentions. Inhale, retain, exhale is half a round; and then another inhale, retain, exhale makes one round. Forty rounds in the morning, forty at midday, forty in the evening, and forty at midnight. A beginner will start with ten or fifteen rounds and then continue until he reaches forty rounds.

During that period you should avoid salty things, as well as pungents, taking mostly sattvic foods such as milk, almonds, cooked rice in milk, ghee, etc. Taking this sattvic food and practicing with yama and niyama, along with the right attitude, will bring purification of the nadis within a few months. Then you will be shining like a bright lotus.

In addition to pranayama practice, you also have to spend time for morning asanas, evening asanas, morning meditation, evening meditation. Then you must have time for bandhas and mudras, study of the scriptures and for singing kirtan. As you must also make time to attend to your natural calls, etc., you might wonder where is the time for sleeping? If you follow this practice, your sleep will come automatically and you won't need much because only one or two hours of sleep will give you perfect rest. Then sleep becomes very deep and undisturbed.

But I am not recommending that you go as fast as that. If you do that now, in your present condition, the kickback will be tremendous. You will be disgusted: "Ugh, I didn't get anything that

Swami mentioned." Start slowly and build up.

I recommend that you practice only three times daily, omitting the midnight practice. You will be getting almost the same benefit without going to that extreme. Really, this is the standard yogic way. When we go into seclusion, this is the way we practice.

If you live in hot climate such as Israel, it is the midday practice which should be omitted. Too much perspiration. Also, I suggest that you avoid extremely cold climates. Some extremists have even practiced pranayama while sitting in the snow, but don't practice this type of pranayama or you will have a complete breakdown of your nervous system. Everything should be moderate: not too cold and not too warm. Moderation is very important.

कनीयसि भवेत्स्वेदः कम्पो भवति मध्यमे।
उत्तमे स्थानमाप्नोति ततो वायुं निबन्धयेत्॥ १२॥

(12) In the first stage (of practice) there is perspiration; in the second, the body feels tremors; in the last, highest stage, the prāṇa goes to the highest spot (Brahmarandhra). Therefore, one should restrain the breath.

There are three stages of purification. The first stage is intense perspiration. When you get perspiration, don't wipe it with your cloth. Instead, rub the sweat into the body with your hand. That sweat is magnetized because of the prana.

In the second [stage], a tremor is felt throughout the body.

The purification continues, and after three or four months of this Alternate Nostril Breathing, Ujjayi, etc., you start Bhastrika. Then the body will show, by way of various signs, that the second stage of purification has been reached. The signs will differ from person to person. The body may start moving so violently up and down that you are unable to control it, indicating that the prana is moving. Some people may experience a tremendous tremor of emotion, others will be more in a still state, some may fall into a kind of swoon, a semiconscious or even an unconscious state. Any of these indicate that the second stage of pranayama has been reached by the yogi who practices yama, niyama and right diet.

Only with these conditions is it good if you enter into this stage. But if you try to create this situation without yama, niyama, right diet, etc., you can rest assured that many reactions will come which you will not be able to control, and nobody will be able to help you. Doctors will not understand. From wrong practice, you might sometimes feel tremendous heat all over the body which a thermometer will not register. Nevertheless, you may feel as if you are on fire. Once in India, a student came up to me and said, "Swamiji, help me, the body is on fire." This was because he was not doing certain things properly, causing these negative reactions to come.

But if the tremor takes place, and if it is the right thing, then you feel at peace inside, and strong. The body may be moving violently but you are peaceful inside. The common reaction is always a blissful inner state. You will want to enjoy that state, to stay in that state. If you get that peaceful experience, you don't have to worry. But when the inner feeling is painful or if it is a negative state, then something is wrong. That is the surest way to find out whether you are progressing or whether you are going in the wrong direction.

> *In the highest stage, the prana goes to the*
> *Brahmarandhra. So one should perform pranayama.*

Randhra means "canal," so Brahmarandhra is "Brahma's Canal." Where is Brahma's Canal? The Sushumna. With this third and highest stage of purification, the tremor will stop and there will be no more perspiration, though your energy is very high. You won't feel anything except the stillness of mind and that inner joy and happiness and peace.

Additional experiences will differ from person to person. Some people may see lights or colors, some may get more vibration in the spinal chord, others won't feel vibration or light anywhere. So if this happens to you, don't think that you are not progressing. These are just individual reactions due to differences in mental states from person to person. When the Kundalini is awakened, outward experiences will differ. These things are not important. The important thing is: are you peaceful? Are you satisfied with your life? Do you know that you are a free man? Do you have the freedom to do what you like now? Are your senses under your control? Is your mind no longer asking you to go to the pizza parlor to find happiness? These are the questions you should be asking. It is the inner experience you should be concerned with, not the external.

Occasionally blockages in the nadis occur as reactions to the taking of drugs, meat, alcohol and so forth, while following this practice. Blocking can take place, not only in the Sushumna nadi, but even in the Ida and Pingala (the normal channels), or in any of the fourteen major nadis, or even in any of the other 72,000 nadis. During blockage prana moves like a wild river, flowing into every nook and corner, going in any direction out of control. At that time it is very difficult to help such people. They never follow instructions, insisting on practicing bandhas, mudras, etc., without adequate preparation. They must first return to normal by changing their diet and other bad practices, and only then can they begin over with simple deep breathing exercises. They should not practice retention in the beginning. Then slowly, slowly as the body becomes normal and the channels purify, then perhaps, after several months they can introduce alternate nostril breathing with retention. But help is very difficult to find for people in such trouble unless they come across a teacher who has had experience of these things and will understand immediately by looking at the person and know how to prescribe.

That is the time when perspiration comes.

The ancients didn't have watches. For them the smallest unit was a matra, which is approximately three seconds. So in the first stage the prana is retained for thirty-six seconds (twelve matras); let us say that it is equal to a half minute.

They used various definitions.

Here they are not talking about physical breathing, but about the prana which is in the Sushumna. When the prana stays in the Sushumna for one and a half minutes, that is called "one breathing," or "one pala." When the prana stays in the Sushumna for more than twelve and a half breathings, it is no longer pranayama, but pratyahara.

There are three stages in the purification of the nadis. In the first stage, perspiration takes place. At the time, the prana is held for twelve matras (approximately 30 seconds). Notice that prana is held, not breath. You hold the prana for thirty seconds in the Sushumna. Prana will not stay for more than a certain time because there is a tremendous resistance there. It's like bringing together the same poles of two magnets: they will repel each other. In the same way, the positive force of the Sushumna and the not-so-purified energy of the Ida and Pingala are coming and pushing against each other. There is a temporary suspension for a very short time. That is called the first stage. So be sure to remember that "thirty seconds" does not mean that we are holding the physical breath. That is what is meant by "holding the breath in the Sushumna."

The second state is held for twenty-four matras. In the third stage, the prana stays in the Sushumna for thirty-six matras (about one and a half minutes), but the true inner feeling of that time appears to be an eternity. Then there is no more time; you are not even aware that the world has any meaning. When you come out of that state, then you know that the world is like a mirage. Don't think that this experience takes place only in the Sushumna. Actually, you feel this radiation throughout your body, and not in a specific location. Location is given only so that your mind can concentrate. It is the same when you focus on chakras so that you can get more concentration power. This helps the energy to flow in the correct channel, which is the most important thing for bringing peace. This is what is meant by "holding the prana" in the different stages.

A word of caution: never take anything literally in Yoga. For example, the symbol of Lord Siva is the dancing Nataraja, representing creation and destruction, the dance of matter. Matter changes every moment. When one particle of matter dies, it becomes new matter for something else. That's called the "Dance of Siva." The petals on chakras are also symbols, hinting at energy pattern radiations. Such things are given so that the mind can visualize. They are just aids for focussing your concentration, so don't get stuck. Use the visualization to come into reality. In reality you never see petals in the chakras.

What you see are the energy pattern changes, the wavelength changes. For at these higher stages of practice you have a different type of experience. These symbols are just aids for focusing your concentration. Many yogic students make the mistake of taking these symbols literally, and when they don't get these experiences, they think that the teachings are all wrong. But that is because they have never approached their teacher to get a proper understanding of them.

In the third stage when certain energies start developing, you may start writing poetry. As the chakras develop, you may see clairvoyantly, or develop various powers, or you may only have the inner peace, not wanting to move, withdrawing from everybody. Reactions will be different, but the inner experience always remains the same: all will have experience of peace and joy.

Again I want to emphasize that we are not talking about the physical breathing but about how long the prana stays in the Sushumna. With twelve and a half palas the prana stays only in the lower chakras, and then at about twenty or thirty palas it goes to the higher chakras. At about 120 palas it reaches the crown. That means that progression in the time of retention will cause the prana to go higher and higher.

Do not expect this to happen in one or two courses or by correspondence, even though it is actually your natural state. It may happen today, tomorrow, or progress might stagnate if you are careless. Now there may be enthusiasm, but if, the moment you finish this Intensive Course, you are tempted by ice cream, pizza, boys and girls, dance and music, and sensual pleasures, then you are finished – the vairagya (dispassion) will be gone. The things you learn from your practice increase your vibratory level; they create a fire. Then it is like taking a glass of water, pouring it over the fire and putting it out.

You will have to start all over again. With fits and starts like this you will not progress very much. What you need is continuous practice. Do not go too fast, such as morning, midday, night, and midnight for three months, and then nothing for three years. If you take that intense an approach there will be a reaction. It is like a man who lifts weights too much and too soon – after five minutes he will have to stop because of aching muscles, and the aching will persist even after he returns home, with the result that he abandons his weight lifting. Also with too much pranayama there will be a mental kickback; the mental pain will be tremendous. Many people are forced to leave the practice because they go too fast and the pain becomes unbearable for them.

This has happened to many students. They go too fast and then hit a roadblock. They stop and then go back to their old rut and stagnate there. In the next life they will have to start all over again, though coming again very quickly to that state where they left off. But if they have not developed viveka and vairagya, they will slip back once more. So, if you are practicing only ten pranayama a day, practice ten pranayama; if you are meditating for half an hour a day, continue. Eventually there will be awakening. If you practice like that – little by little, every day, then the cumulative effect will be much better than a fast few month's work followed by no work at all. Continuous practice is best.

जलेन श्रमजातेन गात्रमर्दनमाचरेत् ।
दृढता लघुता चैव तेन गात्रस्य जायते ॥ १३ ॥

(13) Rub the resulting perspiration on to the body;
as a result, the body is benefited with lightness and
becomes firmer.

In the first stage when you get perspiration, you should rub it well on the body – don't wipe it off. It is a pranic massage when you do that.

अभ्यासकाले प्रथमे शस्तं क्षीराज्यभोजनम् ।
ततोऽभ्यासे दृढीभूते न तादृङ्नियमग्रहः ॥ १४ ॥

(14) In the early stages of practice, food mixed with
milk and ghee is to be taken; but with the
advancement in practice, such restrictions do not
apply.

In the early stages when you are purifying, you must take only food mixed with rice and ghee. You must avoid such things as salt or spices. This you should observe very strictly.

यथा सिंहो गजो व्याघ्रो भवेद्वश्यः शनैः शनैः ।
तथैव सेवितो वायुरन्यथा हन्ति साधकम् ॥ १५ ॥

*(15) As a lion, elephant or tiger is tamed in gradual
fashion, even so should prāṇa be brought under
control gradually. Otherwise it will harm the student
(practicing prāṇāyāma).*

Have you ever seen a tiger in the circus? How are they trained?
Very, very slowly and carefully, watching every evidence of the
cat's moods. And what is the purpose of the chair held in front of
the tiger? It is not only for protection. When the tiger uses his claw
on the chair, the chair doesn't react, and so the tiger, thinking that
the chair is a part of the man's body, is fooled into thinking that
the man is stronger than he is. So even though the tiger is actually
stronger, he is subdued by the man's intellect.

It is the same with the prana. You must try to control the prana
slowly. A violent method, one too fast or without proper diet and
other essential conditions, will cause reactions. Just like an
improperly handled lion or tiger, it will injure you. This stanza is
a warning not to play with prana without following all the rules
and regulations.

प्राणायामादियुक्तेन सर्वरोगक्षयो भवेत्।
अयुक्ताभ्यासयोगेन सर्वरोगसमुद्भव: ॥ १६ ॥

*(16) When prāṇāyāma is practiced diligently as per
rules, one is freed from all diseases. When wrongly
undertaken, many diseases will arise.*

So either you can get rid of all diseases, or you can get all diseases,
depending on how you are practicing.

हिक्काश्वासश्च कासश्च शिर:कर्णाक्षिवेदना:।
भवन्ति विविधा रोगा: पवनस्य प्रकोपत: ॥ १७ ॥

*(17) The defective practice of prāṇāyāma brings
about hiccup, asthama, bronchial diseases, headaches,
earache, eyesore etc.*

Asthma is a breathing difficulty, but this difficulty is not caused by the lungs. It arises because the prana comes to the respiratory system irregularly and also in the wrong direction. The diaphragm or other muscles may be contracting instead of expanding, or the breathing may be too shallow or otherwise incorrect. It is the same with sneezing and coughing – they are nothing but the motion of prana.

Mistaken practices of pranayama which cause disturbances in the prana will cause many types of sickness. That is why you are warned to be careful. The intention is not to frighten you, but to have you practice with care. It is like using a chainsaw; you must know how to operate it or you might cut yourself badly.

युक्तं युक्तं त्यजेद्वायुं युक्तं युक्तं च पूरयेत्।

युक्तं युक्तं च बध्नीयादेवं सिद्धिमवाप्नुयात्॥ १८॥

(18) Exhalation and inhalation should be done in a gradual fashion and the kumbhaka must be done with deliberate steadiness. Only then the haṭhayogī will obtain siddhis.

Not beyond capacity. Only by practicing inhalation, retention, and exhalation in a proportional way do you get control over the prana.

Thus it is that a man obtains siddhis.

यदा तु नाडीशुद्धिः स्यात्तथा जिह्वानि बाह्यतः।

कायस्य कृशता कान्तिस्तदा जायेत निश्चितम्॥ १९॥

(19) When the nāḍīs are pure, definite signs are noticed, such as, leanness of the body and a bright countenance.

You don't feel that the body is heavy. We are not talking about physical heaviness. You will almost feel that you are about to fly all the time (without wings of course). Light and clean. And there is a radiation– the skin, face and eyes all will be radiating and sparkling. This shows that the nadis are purified.

यथेष्टधारणं वायोरनलस्य प्रदीपनम् ।
नादाभिव्यक्तिरोग्यं जायते नाडिशोधनात् ॥ २० ॥

(20) When the nāḍīs are (completely) purified, one can control the breath as desired, the gastric fire (jaṭharāgni) is activated, one can hear the inner sound (anāhata), and there is perfect health.

If the breath is restrained for a longer time (we are not talking about the physical breath), the prana goes into the Sushumna and then there is a balance between the right and the left hemispheres of the brain. Then also both the Ida and Pingala nadis are functioning alternately. That is what is meant by "restraining the breath."

When the gastric fire becomes more active you can eat even poison. Some people hear the nada (inner sounds), others are more likely to see lights, while still others may feel a kind of peace, a silence. Their mind doesn't want to move or hear anything at all – it just wants to rest in that experience of peace or silence. The external experience will manifest differently from person to person, but in all the stages, whether you perceive colors, lights, or sounds, one thing is common to all: the mind is very calm and peaceful. That is the central point which indicates that the nadis are purified. On the other hand, when there is no peace and the mind is constantly wandering, you are unhappy, or in a dejected mood, this shows that the prana is not moving properly because the nadis are purified.

मेद-श्लेष्माधिक: पूर्वं षट्कर्माणि समाचरेत् ।
अन्यस्तु नाचरेत्तानि दोषाणां समभावत: ॥ २१ ॥

(21) Before attempting prāṇāyāma, one who is flabby and phlegmatic should first carry out the six steps or kriyās (as enumerated in śloka 22 below): others who

have achieved balance in their three humors (wind, bile and phlegm) should not do them.

With some people, their nose is running day and night or they are coughing morning and evening. Others are unable to digest food properly because of constant irritation in the stomach. Such people should first practice the six kriyas before beginning intense pranayama. The six kriyas are: Neti, Dhauti, Basti, Tratak, Nauli, and Kapalabhati. (Other kriyas, such as Kunja Kriya, which are long practices, are unnecessary for most people unless they have some specific diseases that call for them.) However, all can benefit from the practice of Jala neti or Sutra neti to keep the nostrils clean. Occasionally you can clean your stomach with salt water and then vomit it out. Kapalabhati, of course, all should practice regularly.

धौतिर्बस्तिस्तथा नेतिस्त्राटकं नालिकं तथा।
कपालभातिश्चैतानि षट्कर्माणि प्रचक्षते॥ २२॥

(22) The six acts are: Dhautiḥ, Bastiḥ, Netiḥ, Trāṭaka, Nauliḥ and Kapālabhātiḥ.

कर्मषट्कमिदं गोप्यं घटशोधनकारकम्।
विचित्रगुणसन्धायि पूज्यते योगिपुङ्गवैः॥ २३॥

(23) These purificatory exercises for the body are to be performed in private. They are held in high esteem by the yogīs because they produce great results.

Such things as the kriyas are not generally given to ordinary people. They are kept secret because they are not meant for public demonstrations.

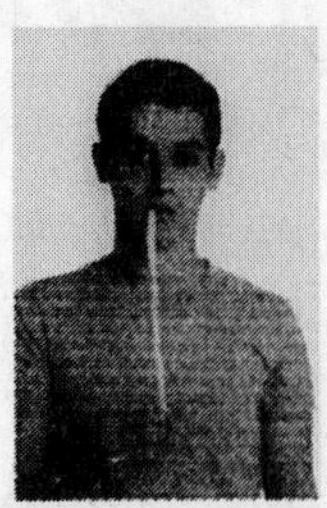

चतुरङ्गुलविस्तारं हस्तपञ्चदशायतम्।
गुरूपदिष्टमार्गेण सिक्तं वस्त्रं शनैर्ग्रसेत्।
पुनः प्रत्याहरेच्चैतदुदितं धौतिकर्म तत्॥ २४॥

(24) Dauṭiḥ (also known as dhauti): Slowly swallow, according to the instructions and guidance of the guru, a wet piece of cloth (thin like muslin), four fingers in breadth and fifteen fingers long. Slowly draw the piece of cloth out. This is the dhauti karma.

कासश्वासप्लीहकुष्ठं कफरोगाश्च विंशति।
धौतिकर्मप्रभावेण प्रयान्त्येव न संशय: ॥ २५ ॥

(25) Dhauti, undoubtedly, is powerful in removing bronchial diseases such as asthama, Plīha (diseases of the glands and spleen and their enlargement), leprosy (and similar skin afflictions) and twenty other diseases brought on by the phlegm. There is no doubt about this.

नाभिदघ्नजले पायौ न्यस्तनालोत्कटासन:।
आधाराकुञ्चनं कुर्यात् क्षालनं बस्तिकर्म तत्॥ २६ ॥

(26) Bastiḥ (also known as basti): Get into water upto the navel and sit in utkaṭāsana resting the body on toes, (and) the heels pressing the buttocks; insert a small bamboo tube into the anus (and contract the anus); this will help draw in water into the stomach; then, shake it (and expel it). This is Basti.

गुल्मप्लीहोदरं चापि वातपित्तकफोद्भवा:।
बस्तिकर्मप्रभावेण क्षीयन्ते सकलामया: ॥ २७ ॥

(27) Practice of Basti helps remove Gulma, Plīha, Udara (dropsy and other stomach diseases) and all

diseases arising from an excess of wind, bile and phlegm.

This is called Basti. When you perform Nauli under these conditions, water is drawn up automatically.

धात्विन्द्रियान्तः करणप्रसादं दद्याच्च कान्तिं दहनप्रदीसिम् ।
अशेषदोषोपचयं निहन्यादभ्यस्यमानं जलबस्तिकर्म ॥ २८ ॥

(28) This jalabasti karma refines bodily dhātus, sense-organs, and internal organs like mind, ego, intelligence etc.; body becomes bright and is able to digest food thoroughly. Many a disorder of the body is cured.

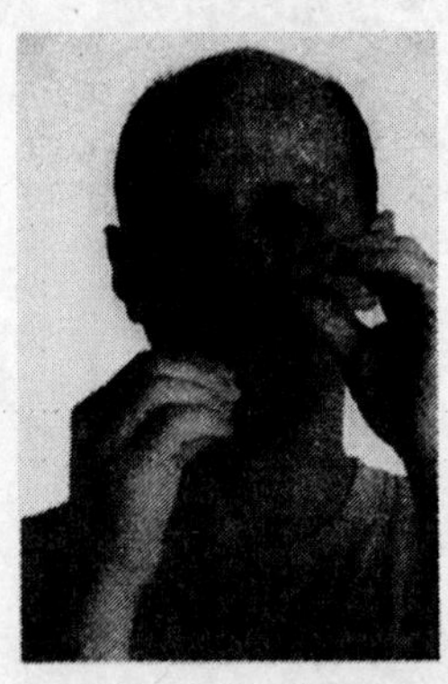

सूत्रं वितस्ति सुस्निग्धं नासानाले प्रवेशयेत् ।
मुखान्निर्गमयेच्चैषा नेतिः सिद्धैर्निगद्यते ॥ २९ ॥

(29) Netiḥ (also known as neti): Insert a nine inches long soft, smooth thread through one nostril and draw it out through the mouth. Siddhas call this netiḥ.

कपालशोधनी चैव दिव्यदृष्टिप्रदायिनी ।
जत्रूर्ध्वजातरोगौघं नेतिराशु निहन्ति च ॥ ३० ॥

(30) Neti purifies the skull and enables the eyes to perceive subtle objects. Also, neti soon removes all diseases of the body above the shoulders.

निरीक्षेत्रिश्चलदृशा सूक्ष्मलक्ष्यं समाहितः।
अश्रुसम्पातपर्यन्तमाचार्यैस्त्राटकं   स्मृतम्॥ ३१ ॥

*(31) Trāṭaka: Look with eyes
(without winking) at a minute
object with concentration till
tears start flowing. This is termed
as trāṭaka by the ācāryas.*

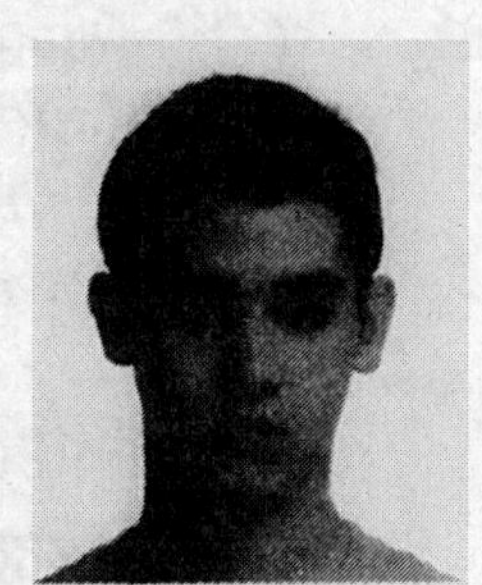

मोचनं नेत्ररोगाणां तन्द्रादीनां कपाटकम्।
यत्लतस्त्राटकं गोप्यं यथा हाटकपेटकम्॥ ३२ ॥

*(32) All diseases of the eyes are removed by
performing trāṭaka; it also gets rid of sloth. It should
be carefully preserved like a golden casket.*

अमन्दावर्तवेगेन   तुन्दं   सव्यापसव्यतः।
नतांसो भ्रामयेदेषा नौलिः सिद्धैः प्रचक्ष्यते॥ ३३ ॥

*(33) Nauliḥ (also known as nauli): With the
shoulders bent down, rotate the stomach right and left
with the speed of a moving eddy. This is called nauliḥ
by the siddhas.*

मन्दाग्निसन्दीपनपाचनादिसन्धापिकानन्दकरी   सदैव।
अशेषदोषामयशोषणी च हठक्रियामौलिरियं च नौलिः॥ ३४ ॥

*(34) Nauli is called the crown of Haṭha-yoga practice;
it stimulates the gastric fire if dull (or slow), increases
the digestive power, produces happiness and destroys
all diseases and disorders of the humors.*

भस्त्रावल्लोहकारस्य रेचपूरौ ससंभ्रमौ।
कपालभातिर्विख्याता कफदोषविशोषणी ॥ ३५ ॥

*(35) Kapālabhātiḥ (also known as kapālabhāti):
Exhale and inhale rapidly like the bellows of a
blacksmith. This destroys phlegmatic diseases. This is
well known as kapālabhātiḥ.*

षट्कर्मनिर्गतस्थौल्यकफदोषमलादिक:।
प्राणायामं तत: कुर्यादनायासेन सिद्ध्यति ॥ ३६ ॥

*(36) These six exercises completely cure obesity,
phlegmatic disorders etc., and remove impurities of a
physical nature. After these (six kriyās) practice of
prāṇāyāma comes effortlessly.*

प्राणायामैरेव सर्वे प्रशुष्यन्ति मला इति।
आचार्याणां तु केषाञ्चिदन्यत्कर्म न सम्मतम् ॥ ३७ ॥

*(37) Some ācāryas say that all impurities of the nāḍīs
are removed by prāṇāyāma alone; the above exercises
are not accepted by them.*

उदरगतपदार्थमुद्वमन्ति प्रवनमपानमुदीर्य कण्ठनाले।
क्रमपरिचयवश्ययनाडिचक्रा गजकरणीति निगद्यते हठज्ञै: ॥ ३८ ॥

*(38) Gajakaraṇī: The eviction of the substances from
the stomach when apāna is drawn up at the throat.
The gradual practice of this act helps control of the
nāḍīs. This is known as gajakaraṇī by those well
versed in Haṭhayoga.*

ब्रह्मादयोऽपि त्रिदशाः पवनभ्यासतत्पराः।
अभूवनन्तकभयात्तस्मात्पवनमभ्यसेत्॥ ३९॥

*(39) Even Brahmā and the other devas regularly do
prāṇāyāma to get rid of the fear of death. Control of
the breath as prescribed is absolutely essential.*

When prana goes to the Sushumna there is no longer any fear at
all.

यावद् बद्धो मरुद्देहे यावच्चितं निराकुलम्।
यावद् दृष्टिभ्रुवोर्मध्ये तावत्कालभयं कुतः॥ ४०॥

*(40) As long as prāṇāyāma becomes a habit and the
mind becomes calm and peaceful, and the eyes are
directed between the eyebrows, why should one fear
death?*

By "breath restrained" is meant that the prana is in the Sushumna.
A mind "firm and steady" is a mind calm and steady. "The eye
directed towards the middle of the eyebrows" does not mean the
physical eye only, but also the mental eye.

विधिवत्प्राणसंयामैर्नाडीचक्रे   विशोधिते।
सुषुम्नावदनं भित्त्वा सुखाद्विशति मारुतः॥ ४१॥

*(41) When the die nāḍī-cakras has been purified by
carefully executed breathing exercises according to the
rules, the breath forces open the mouth of the
suṣumnā and easily enters it.*

At that time prana will go automatically.

मारुते   मध्यसञ्चारे मनःस्थैर्यं प्रजायते।
यो मनःसुस्थिरीभावः सैवावस्था मनोन्मनी॥ ४२॥

(42) The mind becomes peaceful and steady when susumnā is pierced by the breath. This steadiness of the mind is the state called Manonmanī (Unmanī).

Hatha Yoga Samadhi is called Unmani avastha.

तत्सिद्धये विधानज्ञाश्चित्रान् कुर्वन्ति कुम्भकान्।
विचित्रकुम्भकाभ्यासाद्विचित्रां   सिद्धिमाप्नुयात्॥ ४३॥

(43) To attain Manonmanī avasthā, various kumbhakas are performed as laid down; by the practice of various kumbhakas one obtains different siddhis. Now the different types of Kumbhakas:

सूर्यभेदनमुज्जायी सीत्कारी शीतली तथा।
भस्त्रिका भ्रामरी मूर्च्छा प्लाविनीत्यष्टकुम्भका:॥ ४४॥

(44) There are eight kumbhakas viz., Sūryabheda, Ujjāyī, Sītkārī, Śītālī, Bhastrikā, Bhrāmarī, Mūrcchā and Plāvinī.

पूरकान्ते तु कर्त्तव्यो बन्धो जालन्धराभिध:।
कुम्भकान्ते रेचकादौ कर्त्तत्यस्तूड्डियानक:॥ ४५॥

(45) At the end of pūraka the jālandhara-bandha should be practiced. At the end of kumbhaka and at the beginning of exhalation (recaka), uḍḍiyāna-bandha should be practiced.

Jalandhara bandha will block up the prana at one of the most important acupressure areas where various nerves come from. The lungs and the cardiovascular system are both controlled by Jalandhara at the throat. Mula bandha controls the anal sphincter muscles. Jalandhara bandha is practiced as follows: the throat is contracted and the chin firmly placed on the chest.

अधस्तात् कुञ्चनेनाशु कण्ठसङ्कोचने कृते ।
मध्ये पश्चिमतानेन स्यात् प्राणो ब्रह्मनाडिग: ॥ ४६ ॥

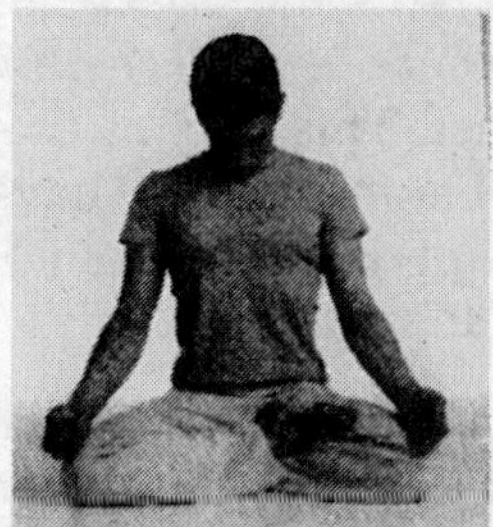

(46) Contracting the throat (i.e., jālandhara-bandha) and the anus (i.e., mūla-bandha) at the same time, and by drawing back the abdomen (in the uḍḍīyāna-bandha) the prāṇa flows through the Brahma nāḍī (suṣumnā).

When both bandhas are applied, the prana flows through the Sushumna for those who are purified through diet and all those things we mentioned. Then prana flows through the Sushumna naturally; it happens automatically without your having to do anything additional about it. Jihva bandha is the tongue lock. If this lock is not known, the anal and chin locks can be practiced without it.

अपानमूर्ध्वमुत्थाप्य प्राणं कण्ठादधो नयेत् ।
योगी जराविमुक्त: सन् षोडशाब्दवयो भवेत् ॥ ४७ ॥

(47) Drawing the apāna forcefully upwards, one should bring the prāṇa downwards from the throat. Then the yogī is freed from old age and becomes a youth of sixteen.

This is apana [downward moving prana]; here its impulse is pulled upward. To get a clear picture of apana, suppose you are driving along a highway and you want to go to the bathroom (your bladder is near to bursting), what do you do? You hold it until you find a toilet, and at that time your bladder is relieved. This control is Mula bandha.

In ancient times, advanced yogis practiced this through Vajroli mudra also (and I am not suggesting that you do it) when they drew water up through the urethra into the bladder with a catheter. It is just like Nauli. This is called "drawing back by the pull of the apana." At first they practiced with water, and then gradually they advanced to the use of milk and honey. Eventually they practiced this in the man-woman union: they could stop the outward flow of the seminal fluid and pull it backwards. Thus the apana for discharging the energy was stopped so that there was no feeling of ejaculation or depression after the sexual act. This tells us that if you know how to control the apana, you will automatically have natural control of moving the sexual energy upwards. This is not part of our practice, but you should have an idea about it.

Those who have difficulties with sexual control can practice Vajroli mudra. This mudra also happens automatically as you contract the anal sphincter muscle in the practice of Mula bandha and also in another mudra called Ashwini mudra, where you sit in water and contract and release the anal sphincter muscles. This practice will help people who have a lack of control such as premature ejaculation or other problems related to the sexual organs. They should, of course, practice this along with the regular practice of pranayama, bandhas and mudras. Then it will become a natural habit for them to draw the apana upwards automatically without any effort. It is a long practice, but like Basti, in time you get full control so that the impulse is withdrawn backwards. Then the apana will not come outwards in the form of a sexual ejaculation.

Apana is used in all sexual acts, in excretion, and also during childbirth. It is apana which is the impulse pushing out the baby. Childbirth is painful because the impulses are coming in an extremely powerful way. A tremendous amount of energy is needed to get the baby out of the mother's womb.

Uddiyana bandha happens naturally when you exhale. In time, with practice, all three bandhas happen automatically.

आसने सुखदे योगी बद्ध्वा चैवासनं ततः ।
दक्षनाड्या समाकृष्य बहिःस्थं पवनं शनै: ॥ ४८ ॥

(48) Sūryabheda: Sitting in a comfortable position and taking up an easy āsana, the student should draw the breath through the (right) piṅgalā nāḍī.

आकेशादानखाग्राच्च निरोधावधि कुम्भयेत्।
ततः शनैः सव्यनाड्या रेचयेत्पवनं शनैः॥ ४९ ॥

(49) (Then) kumbhaka is practiced till prāṇa is felt pervading the entire body head to toe. At the end of kumbhaka, exhale through the left nostril slowly.

कपालशोधनं वातदोषघ्नं कृमिदोषहृत्।
पुनः पुनरिदं कार्यं सूर्यभेदनमुत्तमम्॥ ५० ॥

(50) This sūryabheda kumbhaka should be repeatedly done, as it purifies the brain, destroys diseases arising from the excess of wind (vāta) and cures illnesses caused by intestinal worms.

मुखं संयम्य नाडीभ्यामाकृष्य पवनं शनैः।
यथा लगति कण्ठात्तु हृदयावधि सस्वनम्॥ ५१ ॥

(51) Ujjāyī: Closing the mouth, draw up the breath through the nostrils till the breath fills the space from throat to the heart with a noise.

पुर्ववत्कुम्भयेत्प्राणं रेचयेदिडया ततः।
श्लेष्मदोषहरं कण्ठे देहानलविवर्धनम्॥ ५२ ॥

(52) Perform kumbhaka as before and exhale through idā. This removes afflictions of the throat caused by phlegm and stimulates the fire in the stomach (jatharāgni).

नाडीजलोदराधातुगतदोषविनाशनम् ।
गच्छता तिष्ठता कार्यमुज्जाय्याख्यं तु कुम्भकम् ॥ ५३ ॥

(53) This ujjāyī kumbhaka can be practiced walking or sitting. It removes all defects connected with the nāḍīs and all the dhātus, and dropsy.

The seven dhatus are: skin, flesh, blood, bones, marrow, fat, and semen.

सीत्कां कुर्यात्तथा वक्त्रे घ्राणेनैव विजृम्भिकाम् ।
एवमभ्यासयोगेन   कामदेवो द्वितीयकः ॥ ५४ ॥

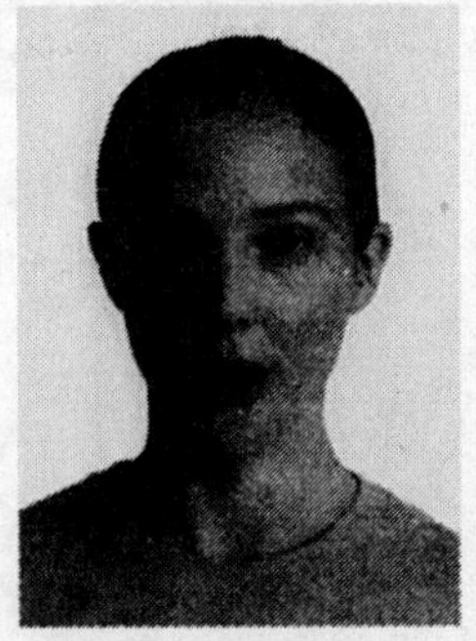

(54) Sītkārī: Place the tongue between the lips and draw the breath in the mouth with a hissing sound and then do the recaka by both the nostril (not by the mouth). Repeating this, one becomes a second god of beauty (second Kāmadeva).

Sitkari differs from Brahmari which has a sound like a bumblebee (very hard). Ujjayi is very mild, very slight. Ujjayi is a major pranayama, while Brahmari, Sitali, and Sitkari are minor pranayamas. A minor pranayama is one which is not very important, but is used for special conditions. For example: Sitali and Sitkari can be used on hot days to cool off the body. They can also be used when the blood is impure or when you wish to stimulate the throat center; the latter is where you cannot get water,

Sitali can be performed as a kind of refrigeration by taking the cool, moist air to the psychic center which creates that thirst.

योगिनीचक्रसंमान्य   सृष्टिसंहारकारक: ।
न क्षुधा न तृषा निद्रा नैवालस्यं प्रजायते ॥ ५५ ॥

(55) Among a gathering of yoginīs, the yogī becomes an object of admiration; he is able to create and destroy; and he is able to control hunger, thirst, sleep and sloth.

He [the author] is giving some kind of chocolate so that people will practice. What this really means is that when there is an abundance of prana, everyone is attracted to your personality. Naturally, when there is honey, honeybees will come. Here the attraction is not due to the body, but to the prana. When there is no prana, you are like a stale pizza. When you have lots of prana like a beautiful fresh rose, people are attracted. Then, as you become older, due to excessive sexual acts, menstruation, gastric problems, lactation, etc., much prana is lost, and then no-one wants to touch you. But if you practice prayanama, there is no old age and so people are attracted to you all the time.

he is able to do and undo; and feels neither hunger, thirst, nor indolence.

This means that if there is food, he will take it. But if he cannot get food at his regular time, he can just take a few deep breaths and stop the hunger impulse. He is not a slave of that particular habit.

भवेत्सत्त्वं च देहस्य   सर्वोपद्रववर्जित: ।
अनेन विधिना सत्यं योगेन्द्रो भूमिमण्डले ॥ ५६ ॥

(56) Verily by this practice a supreme yogī gains strength of body, and remains free from afflictions of every kind on this earth.

जिह्वया वायुमाकृष्य पूर्ववत्कुम्भसाधनम् ।
शनकैर्घ्राणरन्ध्राभ्यां रेचयेत्पवनं सुधीः ॥ ५७ ॥

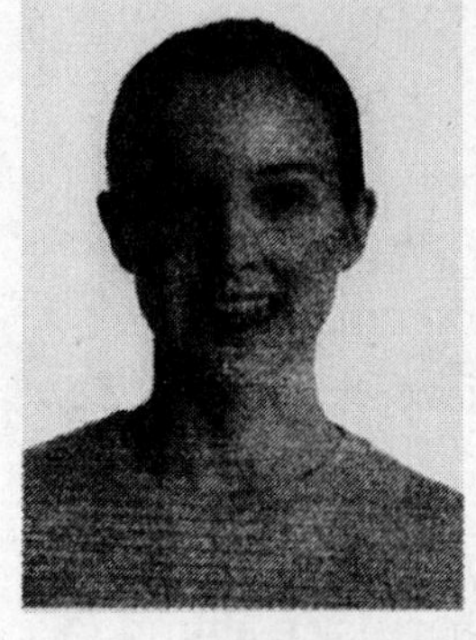

(57) *Śītalī: Protruding the tongue a little away from the lips, curled up resembling a bird's peak, the intelligent one should inhale the prāṇa through the tongue and practice kumbhaka as before and then, should gradually breathe out through the nostrils.*

गुल्मप्लीहादिकान् रोगाञ्ज्वरं पित्तं क्षुधां तृषाम् ।
विषाणि शीतली नाम कुम्भिकेयं निहन्ति हि ॥ ५८ ॥

(58) *This kumbhaka destroys diseases of the abdomen and spleen, fever, bilious complaints, hunger, thirst, and the bad effects of poisons, i.e., snake bites etc.*

ऊर्वोरुपरि संस्थाप्य शुभे पादतले उभे ।
पद्मासनं   भवेदेतत्सर्वपापप्रणाशनम् ॥ ५९ ॥

(59) *Bhastrikā: Place each foot upon the top of the opposite thigh; this is padmāsana which removes all vices.*

सम्यक्पद्मासनं बद्ध्वा समग्रीवोदरः सुधीः ।
मुखं संयम्य यत्नेन प्राणं घ्राणेन रेचयेत् ॥ ६० ॥

(60) *The knowing one sitting firmly in padmāsana with neck and abdomen in one straight line closes the*

mouth and breathes out through the nostrils with force.

यथा लगति हृत्कण्ठे कपालावधि सस्वनम् ।
वेगेन पूरयेच्चापि हृत्पद्मावधि मारुतम् ॥ ६१ ॥

(61) Draw in the breath with a hissing sound till it strikes against the heart; all this time pressure is felt on the heart, the throat and the skull.

पुनर्विरेचयेत्तद्वत्पूरयेच्च पुनः पुनः ।
यथैव लोहकारेण भस्त्रा वेगेन चाल्यते ॥ ६२ ॥

(62) Again, exhaling in the same manner (as mentioned in verse 60) he should draw in the breath and exhale it as directed. Continue this process repeatedly and forcefully with speed, as the blacksmith works his bellows.

This is Bhastrika, which means bellows. You continue like a blacksmith working his bellows until the prana goes to all the chakras. Only if the nadis are first purified from alternate nostril breathing will Bhastrika bring any benefit.

Surya bheda and Ujjayi are heating because they use the right nostril; Sitkari and Sitali are cold. So on hot days you practice Sitali and Sitkari instead of Bhastrika. For the practice of Surya bedha and Ujjayi, you must be in a cool place. Bhastrika uses both nostrils equally, and so is energy-balanced on both sides of the Sushumna. On very hot days, you should omit the practice of Bhastrika during midday; you must be in a cool place for Bhastrika.

तथैव स्वशरीरस्थं चालयेत्पवनं धिया ।
यदा श्रमो भवेद्देहे तदा सूर्येण पूरयेत् ॥ ६३ ॥

(63) *Similarly, keep the prāṇa moving consciously inside the body (by inhalation and exhalation). When tired, one should breathe in by the right nostril.*

यथोदरं भवेत्पूर्णमनिलेन तथा लघु।
धारयेन्नासिकां मध्यातर्जनीभ्यां विना दृढम्॥ ६४॥

(64) *When the breath rapidly fills the stomach, close the nose firmly (with all the fingers, leaving out the middle and index fingers).*

विधिवत्कुम्भकं कृत्वा रेचयेदिडयानिलम्।
वातपित्तश्लेष्महरं शरीराग्निविवर्धनम्॥ ६५॥

(65) *Practising kumbhaka as instructed, breathe out through the left nostril. This removes diseases arising from excess of wind, bile, and phlegm, and increases the digestive fire in the body.*

कुण्डलीबोधकं क्षिप्रं पवनं सुखदं हितम्।
ब्रह्मनाडीमुखे संस्थकफाद्यर्गलनाशनम्॥ ६६॥

(66) *Kuṇḍalinī is roused quickly (by this process). Nāḍīs are purified to a great extent, at the same time experiencing a very pleasant sensation. It removes (destroys) the poison in the form of phlegm etc. at the mouth of suṣumna.*

सम्यग्गात्रसमुद्भूत ग्रन्थित्रयविभेदकम्।
विशेषेणैव कर्त्तव्यं भस्त्राख्यं कुम्भकं त्विदम्॥ ६७॥

(67) Also this bhastrikā kuṃbhaka is essential as it enables the breath to break through the three granthis, or knots, (that are firmly placed in the suṣumnā).

You cannot breat all the granthis at one time. First there is the Brahama granthi of the Muladhara chakra. When the prana and apana unite and the Kundalini awakens, it is this granthi which is broken. Then, as years go by, the prana goes up to the Manipura chakra where the second granthi, the Vishnu granthi, exists. The breaking of this granthi is very difficult, so several lifetimes may be required to break it. The last granthi is the Rudra granthi at the Ajna chakra; when it is broken, the prana goes to the Sahasrara chakra. Bhastrika pranayama breaks these three granthis after purification has taken place, and it is only through Bhastrika that you can break the granthis.

वेगाद् घोषं पूरकं भृङ्गनादं भृङ्गीनादं रेचकं मन्दमन्दम्।
योगीन्द्राणामेवमभ्यासयोगाच्चित्ते जाता काचिदानन्दलीला ॥ ६८ ॥

(68) Bhrāmarī: Inhale rapidly making the sound of a drone (the male bee) and then exhale slowly humming like a bee. By this practice great yogīs derive indescribable joy in their hearts.

पूरकान्ते गाढतरं बद्ध्वा जालन्धरं शनै:।
रेचयेन्मूर्च्छनाख्येयं मनोमूर्च्छा सुखप्रदा ॥ ६९ ॥

(69) Mūrcchā: At the end of the pūraka, practice the jālandhara-bandha firmly and exhale the breath. It reduces mind to a state of inactivity and gives pleasure.

अन्त:प्रवर्त्तितोदारमारुता – पूरितोदर:।
पयस्यगाधेऽपि सुखात् प्लवते पद्मपत्रवत् ॥ ७० ॥

(70) Plāvinī: Having filled the lungs completely with air till they are distended up to the stomach, the yogī is capable of floating effortlessly on deep water (without drowning), like a lotus leaf.

प्राणायामस्त्रिधा प्रोक्तो रेचपूरककुम्भकैः ।
सहितः केवलश्चेति कुम्भको द्विविधो मतः ॥ ७१ ॥

(71) Prāṇāyāma is of three kinds: recaka, pūraka, and kumbhaka is also of two kinds: sahita and kevala.

यावत्केवलसिद्धिः स्यात् सहितं तावदभ्यसेत् ।
रेचकं पूरकं मुक्त्वा सुखं यद्वायुधारणम् ॥ ७२ ॥

(72) Till kevala kumbhaka, which is restraining the breath without pūraka and recaka is achieved, the yogī should practice sahita (kumbhaka).

Sahita kumbhaka is the retention of the regular pranayama with controlled inhalation and exhalation.

For how many years will you continue to practice pranayama? Until you reach Kevala kumbhaka. Kevala kumbhaka is the automatic suspension of breath which occurs when both the right and left nostrils come into balance. Eventually this becomes a natural thing, so that when you sit for meditation the breath stops – just now and then there is an occasional very slow breath through both nostrils.When Kevala kumbhaka is attained, then you can discontinue your practice of pranayama. It takes a long time to attain, but if you continue your practice over the years, it happens. It is similar to the slowing down or stoppage of breath when you are trying to hear something.

When the prana goes in the Sushumna, you can hear the inner sound or feel the peaceful state. When you attain that, you don't

have to continue the intense asanas and pranayama practice –
three or four hours of asanas, pranayama, bandhas, mudras. etc.
are no longer necessary. Just continue with a few asanas and
pranayama so that the body will be healthy and the diagram will
continue to move in the right direction. At that time you should
practice every day only ten or twenty rounds of alternate nostril
breathing, omitting Bhastrika and the other pranayamas. Then you
should try more to hear the inner sound and to keep the prana in
the Sushumna through concentration.

प्राणायामोऽयमित्युक्तः स वै केवलकुम्भकः।
कुम्भके केवले सिद्धे रेचपूरकवर्जिते ॥ ७३ ॥

न तस्य दुर्लभं किञ्चित् त्रिषु लोकेषु विद्यते।
शक्तः केवलकुम्भेन यथेष्टं वायुधारणात् ॥ ७४ ॥

राजयोगपदं चापि लभते नात्र संशयः।
कुम्भकात् कुण्डलीबोधः कुण्डलीबोधतो भवेत्॥ ७५ ॥

*(73) Kevala Kuṃbhaka: This prāṇāyāma when
achieved is known as kevala kuṃbhaka; and it is
devoid of inhalation and exhalation.*

*(74) When this kuṃbhaka is mastered, there is
nothing unattainable in the three worlds; he (the yogī)
is capable of retaining his breath as long as he wants
by the practice of kevala kuṃbhaka.*

*(75) Undoubtedly the yogī also attains the path to
Rāja-Yoga. Kuṇḍalinī is aroused by this kuṃbhaka;
then, due to the arousal of kuṇḍalinī, (suṣumnā
becomes free of all obstacles, and perfection in
Haṭhayoga is obtained.)*

This is called "Chitta vritti nirodha."

Through this kumbhaka, the Kundalini is roused, and when it is so roused, the Sushumna is free of all obstacles and he has attained perfection in Hatha Yoga.

Perfection in Hatha Yoga is perfection in Raja Yoga; they are one and the same.

अनर्गला सुषुम्ना च हठसिद्धिश्च जायते।
हठं बिना राजयोगो राजयोगं बिना हठः।
न सिध्यति ततो युग्ममानिश्ष्पत्तेः समभ्यसेत्॥ ७६ ॥

(76) Suṣumnā becomes free of all obstacles and perfection in Haṭha yoga is achieved. One cannot attain perfection in Rāja-Yoga without Haṭha and perfection in Haṭha yoga without Rāja-yoga; therefore both are to be continuously practiced till their attainment.

This emphasizes the point that one should practice both Yogas simultaneously: asanas and pranayama along with meditation and mantras, not just one Yoga alone.

कुम्भकप्राणरोधान्ते कुर्याच्चित्तं निराश्रयम्।
एवमभ्यासयोगेन राजयोगपदं व्रजेत्॥ ७७ ॥

(77) At the end of kumbhaka, he should withdraw his mind from all objects without exception. When this is continuously practiced, Rāja-Yoga is achieved.

That means pratyahara – don't let the senses go outward.

By thus practicing regularly,
he attains the stage of Raja Yoga.

वपुः कृशत्वं वदने प्रसन्नता नादस्फुटत्वं नयने सुनिर्मले।
अरोगता बिन्दुयोऽग्निदीपनं नाडीविशुद्धिर्हठयोगलक्षणम् ॥ ७८ ॥

इति हठयोगप्रदीपिकायां द्वितीयोपदेशः ॥

(78) The signs of perfection in Haṭhyoga are:
(I) Body becomes lean, (II) Face starts shining,
(III) Clarity in speech or the inner sounds (anāhata
sounds) are heard; (IV) Sight becomes clear, (V) Body
is freed from all diseases, (VI) Seminal fluid is
controlled, (VII) The digestive fire is stimulated, (VIII)
The nāḍīs are purified.

Indicating control of your prana and mind.

the body becomes lean, the speech eloquent,

Although you might not speak grammatically, still your speech is very powerful.

Thus ends the second chapter of *Hatha Yoga Pradīpīka*.

हठयोगप्रदीपिका

Haṭha Yoga Pradīpīkā
CHAPTER THREE

*Kundalini is glorified by all. She Herself, when
awakened by the Yogi, achieves illumination for him.
It is she who bestows liberation and knowledge,
for She is That Herself. She is the source of all
knowledge and bliss. She is pure Consciousness Itself.
She is Brahman, She is Prana Shakti, the Supreme
Force, the Mother of Prana, fire, sound, and the
source of all things.*

- **Swami Sivananda**

SECTION I

INTRODUCTION

Awakening Kundalini

Since most people are content to live only in the lower chakras, their experience of this world is confined to the gross. For example, they may go out to eat in an expensive candle-lit restaurant. Their food is brought by waiters robed in white, carrying elegant covered silver platters. What do they get but the same dog food? (They call it steak.) They sit with a fork and a knife and cut it neatly this way and then put it that way. After eating, they may go to sleep or perhaps go out for a little dancing in order to prepare for a sexual experience later. The next morning they get up just to make money so that they can get power and position to continue this process. They cannot meditate or cogitate: "Who am I? Where do I come from? Where do I go?" One becomes a human being only when these questions begin to be asked, and this happens only when the Kundalini has awakened. Till then, the intellect is used only for the getting of food, sleep, and sensual enjoyments.

Awakening of the Kundalini means that your vibratory level goes up. At that time sensual experience becomes dull and boring; you no longer need drinking, smoking, gambling. It makes no sense to you because you have discovered that satisfaction, peace and happiness are within. Your peace and joy will increase proportionately as this is realized. What ordinary people consider as happiness, is for you nothing but pain. When that experience comes, it means that Kundalini has awakened.

Once the Kundalini is awakened, the fear of death also slowly disappears. Now you know that there is no birth, no death. You find disease vanishing automatically. This is because disease is caused by gross vibrations, by believing that you get happiness from the vibrations of these lower senses. These things will disappear automatically when the Kundalini is awakened.

But don't look for a serpent to come up and hit you. Don't think: "Oh, my Kundalini has reached the third chakra - the fourth chakra - now it is only two more inches to the fifth chakra." That's not the way the Kundalini gets awakened. In actuality, it is the aura condition that changes as the vibratory rate increases.

The highest stage, called God Consciousness, is where the Shakti vibrates with Siva. The lowest stage of Shakti is the experience we get in association with matter. Matter is gross. For example, when your senses come in contact with ice cream, you get an experience of Shakti; it vibrates at a very low level. All of our five senses are Shakti, but they vibrate only when they come in contact with objects, with matter.

When you eat, when you hear music, or when you see something, it excites the Shakti in a very low form. In our lives we are always having such experiences, but we are not happy about them. We want to increase that experience on a different wavelength. So we sit in meditation and try to: (1) quiet the thoughts, (2) regulate the breath, (3) shut off the five organs of action (mouth, speech, legs, hands, genitals and anus), and the five senses of knowledge (hearing, taste, smell, sight and touch). We get knowledge of the universe only through these five senses and we perform actions through the five organs of action. These ten faculties of man are called Indriyas in Sanskrit.

To make the Kundalini Shakti vibrate at a higher level, you must withdraw from contact with external objects. To awaken the Shakti, you must stop the energy from going to the ten faculties so that the mind becomes as still as possible. Then the senses are not reacting on the mind. The mind is not allowed to wander into sensual pathways. Each sense will say, "Come on, let me taste; let me hear," and will draw the mind to the sense objects. But once you are able to stop this extroverted, outward going tendency, you make the mind introverted.

When the mind becomes introverted and still, then the Shakti starts vibrating on a different wavelength. It is awakening to power in a higher state. When the Shakti vibrates only on lower levels, you get only the five basic sensual experiences mentioned above - crude and gross. There is a dissatisfaction with that experience.

You may remember how you used to go for holidays to a five-star hotel. Early morning you drank coffee, you smoked, you ate your breakfast with bacon and eggs, and then swallowed a couple of aspirins or pep pills. Afterwards you sat by the swimming pool or went to the golf course or went fishing. In the evening you ate your steak and then you went dancing. The senses went only in this direction; you never knew anything beyond that. But now you are looking for something else because you are unhappy living at the low energy level like that of an animal. You want to get out of the animal experience to a divine experience.

The ordinary human experience is very close to animal experience and perhaps even worse, because we become very clever at using the intellect to satisfy the senses: how to alter the natural flavor of food by cooking and spicing so that it will taste better, or how to combine it with certain drinks so that it will be even more tasty. In this way you use the intellect to prepare food, spending hours and hours in changing its nature so that it will have a different flavor and appearance. All the senses are brought into action - that is why there is unhappiness and pain in all of us. That pain has brought you to this point.

But the Raja Yoga we are stopping the outgoing senses and stilling the mind. Raja Yoga is called "Citta vritti nirodha," stopping the mental waves. In Hatha Yoga we stop the pranic waves so that the mental waves will stop. In Kundalini Yoga they say that when the senses are brought together, the energy will not move outward. At that time, thought will be in a higher vibratory level; the energy field will change. Actually, all these experiences are one and the same, only the point of view is different. There is really no difference between Kundalini Yoga, Hatha Yoga, Mantra Yoga, Laya Yoga, and Raja Yoga. Each Yoga may emphasize certain points, but they are not basically different from each other. They are all part of Ashtanga Yoga (the eight-limbed Yoga): yama, niyama, asana, pranayama, pratyahara, dharana, dhyana and samadhi.

Mantra Yoga achieves energy/thought control by the use of mystic syllables. When you repeat "On Namo Narayanaya" over and over again, you are changing the vibratory level of your thought. In Kundalini Yoga, by pulling the energy upward through control of the prana, the energy field changes its wavelength. In Hatha Yoga, by controlling the prana, the Kundalini is pushed upward, and in this way too the energy level is changed. So you may say that eventually all these techniques are nothing but Kundalini Yoga.

The Shakti must be controlled and transformed into a higher vibratory state.

When You perform asanas, you are not just performing physical exercise. Asanas also act on the psychic system (just as acupuncture affects the various meridians) by stimulating the prana. For example, when there is a problem in the liver, acupuncturists stimulate the appropriate area of a meridian with a needle so that the electrical impulses increase and the liver gets additional prana for its healing. But yogis can do the same without the need for needles, just from the asanas themselves. Take a Kirilian photograph before you do asanas and another one afterwards. You will see that the energy level has changed completely with a tremendous new emanation of energy. This has been proven by recent scientific research.

And when you perform pranayama, not only do you get oxygen, but the wavelength of the chakras (the energy field) changes. This is being investigated by Eastern as well as Western scientists. In Japan, researches have a chakra machine which can actually measure the energy wavelength in each chakra. It is like an especially sensitive microphone which picks up the wavelength radiating from each chakra without even touching the body. The signal is then passed through an amplifier and into an oscilloscope so that the wave pattern can be viewed. Each chakra will be seen to show a different wave pattern. When advanced yogis meditate, their chakras vibrate rapidly and so the pattern in the oscilloscope changes. Before this recent research, we had no way to prove the existence of these human energy fields.

This shows that Kundalini Shakti is manifesting in a higher dimension. The purpose of all this pranayama is to increase the vibratory level or awaken the Kundalini Shakti - they are one and the same. That is why we use various methods: physical, mental and pranic. The physical method is by controlling the sphincter muscle of the anus, by applying Jalandhara bandha to affect the vagus nerve. When both impulses are controlled, the energy builds up.

It is like the electronic flash on a camera. When you turn on the flash, energy from the six-volt battery builds up in the condenser little by little. Then when you press the button, a flash of light comes (about 10,000 - 20,000 volts for a fraction of a second) to take the photograph. This flash is very intense and powerful, so you get a tremendous amount of light, even though for only a fraction of a second. The same thing happens when you hold the breath and control the energy.

As you hold the breath, you lower batteries start charging up - with both prana and apana. Then suddenly, one day when the nadis are purified, the energy starts flashing through the spinal cord in an instant. At that time all of the chakras are opened up. This is the awakening of the chakras by the movement of the kundalini to the asanas, pranayama, and purification by chanting mantras and eating right diet–the energy must go up automatically. Your spiritual progress will increase proportionally as the energy level goes to the "awakening of the Kundalini Shakti."

This should be understood theoretically. The energy is within you; it is to be awakened. Do not make it grosser or bring it to a lower state. Withdraw the senses as much as you can and bring that energy to the higher centers through your imagination and concentration. Wherever you think, there the prana goes; that is a law. Conversely, wherever prana goes, there thought goes. Thought and prana are interrelated; one cannot move without the other also moving.

That is why concentration, imagination, and physical exercise together give you a complete holistic approach to the awakening of the Shakti. That is why you need asanas, pranayama, bandhas, mudras, right diet, and the right atmosphere. A right atmosphere would be beautiful mountains where the magnetic current (the prana) is very strong from all the vegetation. Everything in nature radiates so that you can absorb and store this prana for your higher spiritual development.

PRANA AS ELECTRICITY

Your physical body is like a machine. It runs on two types of energy: chemical energy, which comes from food, and psychic energy (called prana) which comes from all the objects we take in: food, water, air, and sunlight. These are the basic sources of our prana, and they are found everywhere in nature. Prana also exists in the vacuum of space, underground, and even in water. But it is not a chemical thing, it is electrical in nature. Your body is a storehouse of prana, and the blood system [circulatory system] acts as a transformer, diverting the prana from the astral to the physical.

Yogis do not believe that the body exists merely because of its physicochemical nature; to then it is basically electrical in nature. When the electrical connection from the astral to the physical is severed (like a battery disconnected from an engine), it doesn't matter how powerful the engine is, it cannot start. The impulses of prana travel through the astral to the physical through an astral umbilical cord at our solar plexus. When this cord is severed, no more prana can come to the physical body. If the prana comes in very small amounts then the body will be comatose (unconscious).

If you understand the electrical nature of our bodies, you will understand the purpose of pranayam. I will try to explain in modern terms, as some of the ancient terms are very difficult to grasp.

It is said that you can block the air in the Sushumna, in the throat region, in the stomach region, in the back region, in the ear region, in the eye region. Actually, how can you block the air in these places when the air which you inhale does not go into these places at all? What does this mean?

Actually, it is not a physical blockage, it is the diversion of energy from one source to another. In Yoga we call this energy "prana." The problem is that there is no English equivalent for this word, so it gets translated as "air." Even Indian yogis make this mistake when they don't know how to translate from the Sanskrit.

I like to explain these ideas using analogies with electronic terms. Most of you are familiar with such gadgets as radios, cameras, computers. There are three basic components common to all of them.

Similar things exist in your body, but please don't take what I say literally; it is only to help you to understand how such things as locks work in the body mechanism. When you do pranayama, it will help you a great deal if you understand this. Three things should be understood: (1) transformers, (2) condensers, and (3) resistors.

(1) **Transformers**: In electronic components there is always a source of power, usually a battery or household current. A small tape recorder cannot handle the 110 volt current as it enters the house, so it must be stepped down to a lower voltage by a transformer, otherwise the components will burn up. (There are step-down transformers and step-up transformers for decreasing and increasing the voltage.)

(2) **Condensers** (also called **Capacitors**) are storehouses of electricity. An example is the electronic flash in your camera. The electricity for the flash may come from a six volt battery, but that voltage cannot give enough light to take a photograph. What is needed is several thousand volts to create an intense light. So the energy coming from this small battery is stored up (it is not stepped up or stepped down) like a reservoir and accumulated till it can create a powerful flash for a brief moment.

(3) **Resistors**: Another concept in electronics that we should understand is that of resistance. We can increase or decrease the resistance to the flow of energy. More impurities will reduce the electrical flow. An example is the ordinary garden hose through which water flows at a specific velocity unless constricted by squeezing. The pump continues to try to force 16 gallons of water per minute through the hose, but when its capacity is reduced by constriction, the pressure goes up, and so the water comes out more forcefully.

In our body, something similar to a condenser also exists. Prana is like electricity but very subtle. All electricity flows through wires, and in our body it flows through nadis (or meridians in the Chinese system). The problem here, is that when I say nerve, many people understand only the visible type of nerve. The nadi is equivalent to the nerve in the physical body, but it may be called an astral nerve tube, as it exists not in the physical, but in the astral body. I will not be able to completely communicate this subject in electronic terms, but there does exist a similarity between a physical nerve and your astral nerve; they are counterparts. The difference is that one is visible and the other is not.

In our bodies, the impulse coming from the brain through the vagus nerve which controls the heart and lungs are all impulses called prana. Previously it was thought that the heart was not susceptible to voluntary control, that you could not control the heartbeat by concentration. But yogis can demonstrate that the heartbeat can be slowed down with concentration or by such practices as Jalandhara bandha. They shut down the flow of prana. We are not talking about physical prana, but psychic prana.

Thought can change your breathing rhythm as well as your heartbeat. Two important components of the body are together called the cardiovascular system because they are interdependent. When the body needs extra oxygen, the heart rate goes up. In order to make the lungs pump faster you have to stimulate the muscles of the diaphragm and intercostal muscles. That is done by the brain. In an emergency, say you are running because a tiger is chasing you and you are close to exhaustion, the adrenal glands will throw out adrenaline to give the heart an extra boost so that the lungs can breathe a bit faster for a short time. That's equivalent to the capacitor in electronic gadgets which I mentioned. Nature has given us this ability to escape from dangerous situations. This extra stimulation activate the adrenal gland which pumps adrenaline into the blood stream so that the heart gets a fast kick for a short time so that it can pump more oxygen to the muscles. Let us try to understand the cardiovascular system, to see how the heart rate and the breathing are interconnected.

There is a gadget called the polygraph or lie detector. Just as EEG tests the brain waves, the polygraph measures the three basic components mostly connected to the autonomous nervous system, a system which is basically not under our control. Generally speaking, the autonomous nervous system is beyond our control, but yogis can control it. In the polygraph, the three basic components are: (1) to demonstrate and measure your breathing pattern, how many cycles per second you are breathing (normally we breathe 16 times per minute); (2) the pulse rate (normally about 75 or 80 per minute); (3) galvanic skin response. Under our sweat glands there are nerves which carry sensory impulses.

Because the galvanic skin response (GSR), measured as coming from the sweat gland, will change according to your thought, it is one of the three basic components in a polygraph. When you check for GSR by putting small electrodes on the tip of the finger (for example), you can take this current coming out and amplify it so that you can see its pattern. That is also under the autonomous nervous system.

The polygraph technician also connects and elastic type of material from your chest to the polygraph so that you can see the number of times you are breathing, or what your breathing pattern is: shallow, long, or disturbed. With normal breathing we inhale about 1500 cc of air and exhale out the same amount very gently. But when you are breathing deeply, you can take in and out about 2000 cc. At that time the impulse will be very strong. When you are mentally disturbed the breathing pattern will also change.

When all these components are connected to the polygraph, we observe three different waves: breathing pattern, blood pressure, and galvanic skin resistance. After two or three minutes there is a normal reading. If suddenly the polygraph changes, it is an indication that the person has lied. An emotional upset will cause the breathing pattern to change from say sixteen times per minute to twenty-five or thirty times per minute. It can go up or down. In extreme cases the breathing or the heart may even stop, as in the case of shock or some bad news. Also good news: something very exciting - say you won five million dollars in a lottery - that could stop the heart also.

In such cases you are overloading your capacitor. Within a brief time, everything is short circuited. The voltage coming through the nerves becomes so powerful that it just short circuits everything: the heart and/or lungs stop and there is collapse. So you see that your body is not different from an electronic mechanism.

The electronic impulse in our body is the prana. This prana comes to the nervous system where it is stored by condensers and transformed by transformers. There are five basic types of prana: prana, apana, udana, samana, and vyana, as well as some minor pranas; the difference between major and minor pranas lying in the voltage. Even in electronic gadgets, some things need higher voltage so there are different types of transformers. [In the body] we call these transformers chakras. Various nerves come and go through the chakras. They are not physical nerves, but astral.

In the physical body, the places where these nerves gather at the spinal cord are called plexuses. They are a kind of junction like a telephone exchange. These plexuses correspond to the chakras. This is where the energy is stored up like a condenser, altered like a transformer and acted upon by resistors. All these things take place in the same area.

In most people, the transformers in their upper chakras are not completely opened up; maybe for highly advanced students they are partially opened. Or if there is a tremendous amount of impurity, it acts as a resistor. These variable resistors are automatically controlled by your thought [as well as your diet]. Everything is controlled by thought. According to the nature of your thought, your impurities will increase or decrease. For each of these three gadgets in your system: condenser, transformer, resistor, all are controlled by your mind.

So yogis go directly to the mind to change the pattern. According to the nature of the pattern of your thought, the voltage will be increased or reduced. If the voltage increases, then the energy goes to a higher chakra. If you reduce the voltage (make your thought very gross with only sensual and sexual thoughts), then the energy goes only to the lower chakras because the voltage is not sufficient to lift to the higher chakras.

Remember that neither thought nor prana are in the physical body. They are in the astral body and according to the nature of your thought, the prana flows in the physical body. When your thought is very gross, then the prana or electrons coming to the physical body will be lessened since there is too much resistance. Also, a physical nerve cannot take a high, powerful thought, so there may be a shutdown of the prana to a certain extent. The nervous system which is impure cannot transmit high voltage. Sometimes a sudden shock to the mind will even shut off this flow of prana. Sometimes this current is slowed down to such an extent that you are like a living corpse. Then you are in a coma.

BANDHAS AND MUDRAS

Bandhas are locks; they lock the prana in a certain area. Mudras are seals; they seal certain things and cause the energy to flow in only one direction instead of alternately. Again, we have to go back to electronics to understand these things.

You all now understand about resistance. Another thing to consider is alternating current (AC) and direct current (DC). The light bulbs in our homes work off alternating current because the positive and negative poles change as the dynamo rotates. On the other hand, direct current (DC), such as the current from a battery will light such gadgets as a flashlight. With DC, the flow of electrons is not alternating; it comes in steady streams.

When we apply the seals (mudras) and locks (bandhas), we are allowing the electrons to flow in only one direction (not alternately), and we are stopping the afferent and efferent currents (the motor and sensory impulses). In this way, the normal pattern of energy throughout the nervous system is altered. Through bandhas, mudras and pranayama, we control the sensory and motor nerves.

If you regularly practice the above (with purification of the nadis), then the energy will flow through one channel, the Sushumna, like direct current. This gives a high voltage, less resistance and more capacitance. When you have all these put together in an electronic component such as the electronic flash, the capacitor is charged and voltage builds up until there is an intense discharge of bright light for a fraction of a second. Too much resistance will cause everything to blow up because the flow through that wire must be sufficient to accommodate all those electrons. So we must remember the concepts of resistance, a build-up of voltage, and eventual discharge.

This also happens in our sexual experience. The capacitors are charged from thoughts and passion, and then in the sexual climax, suddenly there is a discharge of the prana. Afterwards there is no energy for you. You all know how the sexual act (or any strong emotion such as anger) literally drains the body of energy. After discharge takes place, it takes several hours to recharge the capacitors. It is just like an electrical flash: you can't press the discharge button immediately and get light again, you have to wait to build up the charge once more. That is why after the sexual act you have to wait for the body to recharge. A man who goes on wasting this energy, one day will become impotent like a dead battery. Then there is no happiness in him, no peace of mind. It's not just physical impotence I'm talking about - there will also be mental impotence. Thought becomes dull; one becomes unable to properly channel thought currents, and emotional complications take place, resulting in constant depression. All of this happens due to excessive discharge of prana.

Western scientists do not properly understand this. They think that the sexual act is a natural thing. It is not. It needs a tremendous amount of charging of the capacitors, and then there is release of heat energy in a very short time. Suppose you were to continually discharge the flash on your camera after each build up of the capacitor, soon the battery would become so completely discharged that you would have to replace it. However, in our bodies we cannot change the battery; we have to wait while we recharge normally or do pranayama. Ordinary people do not know what pranayama is, so they can recharge only through rest, sunshine and eating food. You get some prana from eating food, but it is a very little bit: just the minimum amount for survival and the carrying on of vegetative functions.

Ordinary people cannot do higher practices of meditation, thinking, higher willing. Even though they may be doctors, psychiatrists, PhDs, they don't even have enough willpower to stop their smoking habits as their higher psychic capacities are very limited. They are continuously discharging and they don't know how to recharge. Their mind is in a very weak condition. If you understand this, they you understand the purpose of bandhas and mudras.

From practicing pranayama along with the bandhas and mudras, you are slowly channelling the current into one direction. Normally your energy is oscillating, like alternating current. As you channel the energy into one current, your capacitors charge up. Each time you hold the breath, you are recharging the capacitors. As each chakra transformer pulsates, the voltage increases and goes to higher and higher chakras. As the voltage goes up, each chakra acts like a step-up transformer, increasing the energy level step by step until the energy reaches the Sahasrara. This is called union.

This is the theory behind Kundalini Yoga. In philosophical terms, the aim of spiritual practice is freedom from mundane life into divine life. In Kundalini terms, this freedom or Mumukshutva is actually an escape from the lower voltage to a higher voltage.

SECTION II

सशैलवनधात्रीणां   यथाधारोऽहिनायक: ।
सर्वेषां योगतन्त्राणां तथाधारो हि कुण्डली ॥ १ ॥

(1) Kuṇḍalinī is the main support of all yogic sādhanas like the Lord of serpents, Ananta, bears aloft the whole terra firma with all the mountains and trees.

सुप्ता   गुरुप्रसादेन यदा जागर्ति कुण्डली ।
तदा सर्वाणि पद्मानि भिद्यन्ते ग्रन्थयोऽपि ॥ २ ॥

(2) When Kuṇḍalinī which lies dormant and inactive is aroused by the guru's grace, then, all the cakras (lotuses) and granthis (knots) are pierced.

The granthis are in the Sushumna. The Brahma Granthi is in the Muladhara Chakra, the Vishnu Granthi in the Manipura Chakra, the Rudra Granthi in the Ajna Chakra. They can be broken by practicing pranayama, bandhas and mudras.

What is meant by "the grace of the guru?" If you have faith in the guru, he will teach you when you are ready to practice.

प्राणस्य   शून्यपदवी तद   राजपथायते ।
तदा चित्तं निरालम्बं तदा कालस्य वञ्चनम् ॥ ३ ॥

(3) Prāṇa gets an easy passage through the suṣumnā nāḍī. Then, the mind remains suspended and the yogī conquers Time (death).

सुषुम्ना शून्यपदवी ब्रह्मरन्ध्रं महापथ: ।
श्मशानं शाम्भवी मध्यमार्गश्चेत्येकवाचका: ॥ ४ ॥

(4) Suṣumnā, Śūnyapadavī, Brahmarandhra, Mahāpatha, Śmaśāna, Śāmbhavī and Madhyamārga are synonymous.

This is difficult to understand, though if you are practicing you will understand a little bit. "The void" is a literal translation from the Sanskrit "shunya," meaning no quality, no time or space or awareness. So, when the prana goes into the Sushumna, the world becomes non-existent. Time awareness, space awareness, experiences of the senses are only created by the mind, by thought. Ordinarily, sometimes you are active and sometimes you are not; you have bad emotions, good emotions - this goes on constantly. Then there are qualities and you are aware of space and time. But once prana reaches the Sushumna, it becomes void. In other words: samadhi is attained.

In Hatha Yoga we call this state Unmani avasta. In Raja Yoga it is called Asamprajnata samadhi. In Bhakti Yoga it is called Bhava samadhi. In Jnana Yoga this state is called Nirvikalpa samadhi. But they are all the same thing.

Brahmarandhra means Brahma's Canal. At present, prana goes through Ida and Pingala (through sensual and sexual organs), but when it goes through the Brahmarandhra you will be thinking, "Aham" - "I Am."

Samadhi is also called "burning ground." What are you burning? You are burning all your samskaras (subtle impressions from past lives) which, though hidden, will sprout like seeds in the springtime. When the prana goes into the Sushumna they are burnt.

तस्मात्सर्वप्रयत्नेन प्रबोधयितुमीश्वरीम् ।
ब्रह्मद्वारमुखे सुसां मुद्राभ्यासं समाचरेत् ॥ ५ ॥

(5) Therefore, the yogī should carefully practice the various mudrās to wake up the great Goddess (Kuṇḍalinī) which lies asleep at the entrance of the Brahmarandhra.

महामुद्रा महाबन्धो महावेधश्च खेचरी।
उड्यानं मूलबन्धश्च बन्धो जालन्धराभिधः ॥ ६ ॥

करणी विपरीताख्या वज्रोली शक्तिचालनम्।
इदं हि मुद्रादशकं जरामरणनाशनम् ॥ ७ ॥

(6 and 7) The ten mudrās listed here destroy old age and death: They are Mahāmudrā, Mahābandha, Mahāvedha, Khecarī, Uḍḍīyāna, Mūlabandha, Jālandhara-bandha, Viparītakaraṇī, Vajrolī, and Śakticālana.

Khechari is the cutting of the tongue. It brings an artificial type of samadhi called Jada samadhi, or inert samadhi; it cannot bring you the highest experience or destroy your desires. It is a way of trying to stop the prana without purification.

Vajroli is the physical contraction which draws water up through the urethra. Then one gradually increases the density of the liquid (by using honey, etc.) so that eventually even a sexual ejaculation can be withdrawn backwards. It is similar to Basti, where water is drawn up into the colon by the vacuum created from performing Nauli. But for our purposes it is not necessary to practice Vajroli because we can get these benefits from Mula bandha by stopping the very impulse.

Uddiyana, Mula and Jalandhara bandhas you already know.

Viparita karani is like the shoulderstand but in a slanting position. Its purpose is to bring the energy backwards. Generally the nectar is dripping from the moon in the upper area and the sun below is swallowing it all the time. But by inverting the body, this nectar is caught, and then the body remains youthful. That's the theory behind it. Viparita karani should be practiced only in the morning, not in the evening.

To do Shakti chalani, you perform Bhastrika and then you bounce the body up and down.

Before practicing any of these mudras and intense pranayama, you definitely must be very careful about your diet. You also cannot indulge too much in uncontrolled sexual practices as this will bring prana in the wrong direction. So practice celibacy as much as you can, but don't suppress sex; sublimate it. Practice yamas and niyamas, do lots of japa for purification. Then Shakti gets awakened by Shakti chalani like a ripe fruit which is very tasty. But when you take unripe fruit and try to beat it to make it ripe, it may appear to be soft, but it will be sour. The same is true with all spiritual practices. Let it ripen, don't be in a hurry.

> *these are the ten mudras that destroy old age and death.*

Death and old age may be there, but you are not afraid of them since they pertain only to the physical body. There are many siddhas still around who can move about in both the physical and astral worlds. When they come to the physical world, they can take the physical pattern and convert it into a physical body so they can appear before their students. Or if they want to go to other dimensions they can wander around without visa or passport. Saint Narada is an example. He just uses his veena, sings "Om Namo Narayanaya," and he goes to whichever plane he wishes to travel. Sometimes he also comes to the earth plane.

आदिनाथोदितं दिव्यमष्टैश्वर्यप्रदायकम् ।
वल्लभं सर्वसिद्धानां दुर्लभं मरुतामपि ॥ ८ ॥

> *(8) These divine mudrās are created by the great primeval Lord Śiva and by practicing them yogīs gain the eight siddhis; these siddhis are sought after by all siddhas and are difficult to obtain even for the Maruts (devas).*

There are eight [psychic] powers [or siddhis]. But they are not the purpose of your practice – remember that. They come to test you to see whether the mind is weak or strong. It is very easy to be tempted. If you get these siddhis and you demonstrate them once or maybe twice, then they leave you. Siddhi means energy like electricity, due to the power built up in the various chakras. If you have a battery, you can use it for lighting or anything, but when it is used up, it is dead.

So if the siddhis come, you are really in a dangerous situation because temptation will be very great. All power corrupts, that is the law. Siddhis are just a distraction for the mind; the prana may be accumulating, but using siddhis just disperses the prana. Perhaps it took you several lives to reach a certain level, but just for a few minutes of pleasure by using siddhis, you fall down to the bottom and have to start all over again. It is just not worth it. Create siddhis but don't worry about them; they are not your goal. Anyway, they usually come only when you don't want them. Sivananda had the eight siddhis, but he never demonstrated them; he always prostrated before everybody.

They are much sought after by all siddhas, and are difficult to obtain even by the devas.

Even angels in heaven cannot obtain these powers because they don't have a physical body. They have an astral body. As they live on the astral plane, they can't create fresh karma. They live only in heaven with the karma which they created in their past lives. They have to wait for thousands of years before they come back to the planet – again get a human body, again find a good teacher, and again start to practice. They may not even start, because as they are still living in the pleasure centers in heaven, when they come back, they may just be born in say, New York City, where they know only champagne and caviar.

That is why angels are afraid of yogis like you who are practicing and disciplining your life. They are jealous because you go beyond them, so they put obstacles in front of you. They try to tempt you with various types of powers, but they are all obstacles.

गोपनीयं प्रयत्नेन यथा रत्नकरण्डकम् ।
कस्यचिन्नैव वक्तव्यं कुलस्त्रीसुरतं यथा ॥ ९ ॥

(9) This should be carefully kept secret as a casket of precious diamonds. It should not be divulged to

> *anyone – just as the liaison with a married woman of noble family.*

The three basic locks and seals are Maha bandha, Maha mudra and Maha vedha. They are very simple to learn, but the Pradipika says to keep them secret – do not give them to everybody. First of all, people will laugh when they hear such things. They won't understand what it means to get the breath into the Sushumna. So do not talk about this to anybody unless they are qualified through practice. Then benefit will come from these three beautiful practices.

At this point I want to talk about the nature of prana and its motion. As the body is not only chemical in its nature, but also electrical, yogis can operate on the electrical body (the energy body) through pranayama, bandhas, and mudras. These operations are all interrelated.

In the beginning of your practice, you tried to purify the nadis through Anuloma Viloma (alternate nostril breathing) with a proportion of 1:4:2. You did this so that the prana (the impulse of life force coming from the brain) might come to a kind of rhythm. (Eventually you can also have rhythm of the apana, but only when you have practiced for a very long time.)

What you discover is not a physical thing, as mudras and bandhas are more subtle than asanas or pranayama. Even a beginner can see the benefits of asanas. Asanas and pranayama operate more on the gross physical level, but they are the road to the mudras and bandhas.

What is called meditation in Raja Yoga, is called "stopping the impulses" in Hatha Yoga. But they are one and the same. If you want to stop the fan, you must turn off the switch so that the electrical impulse will no longer reach the motor which drives the blades. Likewise, what we are trying to do is to turn off the switches to various senses through the power of thought.

Prana accumulates while breathing very gently. At that time, application of the bandhas causes the heartbeat to go down. Also the pulse rate slows down, metabolic activity slows down, and brain waves go down from beta to alpha. With even greater control of the breath, the brain waves go down to the theta stage (three to seven cycles per second), and then eventually they stop. So we see that the brain waves change according to the breathing quality.

What we are trying to do with bandhas and mudras is simple to understand. In everyday life we select from among the many sounds we hear as we focus mainly on the sounds which are pleasing to us and try to block unpleasant ones. Examples might be the sound of a jackhammer breaking up a road, or the sound of someone scolding us. We try to block such impulse so that they do not go to the brain and create a negative sensation in the thought atmosphere. We do the same with a horrible sight or with a bad smell such as a skunk odor. We try to shut these off. In the same way, with bandhas and mudras, we are just switching off the impulses going to the brain. We may not be able to shut off everything, but we try to stop as much as possible. In the beginning we have to learn to control by individual "switches," but later on it becomes so habitual that we can just use "remote control." Everything comes to a standstill.

Perhaps you think that some great teacher will touch you and you won't have to practice any asanas, bandhas or mudras. It doesn't usually happen this way; only in rare cases it can happen because of the student's practice of these things in past incarnations. If many of his blocks are gone, the few that remain in the present incarnation can be removed by even a teacher's gaze, a touch, or a word. Then the student reaches the highest samadhi. But as I said before, this is very rare.

पादमूलेन वामेन योनिं सम्पीड्य दक्षिणम् ।
प्रसारितं पदं कृत्वा कराभ्यां धारयेद् दृढम् ॥ १० ॥

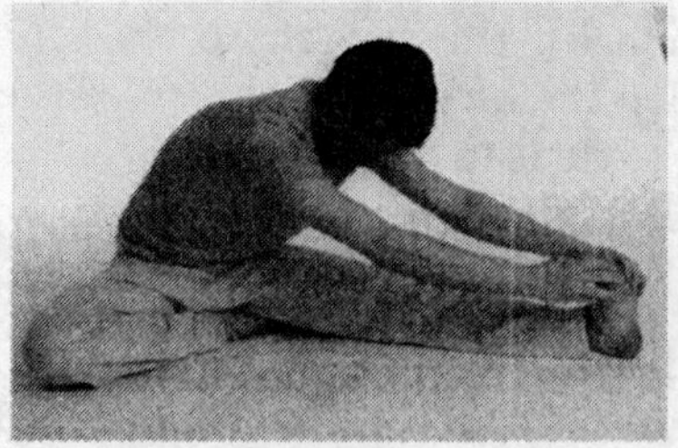

(10) Pressing the perineum with the left heel and stretching out the right leg, take firm hold of the toes (of your right foot) with both hands.

कण्ठे बन्धं समारोप्य धारयेद्द्युमूर्ध्वतः।
यथा दण्डहतः सर्पो दण्डाकारः प्रजायते॥ ११॥

(11) Then contract the throat (in the Jālandhara-
bandha) and hold the breath in the upper part (i.e.,
in the suṣumnā). Then the kuṇḍalinī becomes straight,
just as a coiled snake when struck by a rod suddenly
straightens itself like a stick.

ऋज्वीभूता तथा शक्तिः कुण्डली सहसा भवेत्।
तदा सा मरणावस्था जायते द्विपुटाश्रया॥ १२॥

(12) Then, Kuṇḍalinī becomes straight at once. Then
the two other nāḍīs (iḍa and piṅgala) become dead,
because the breath goes out of them.

ततः   शनैः शनैरेव रेचयेन्नैव वेगतः।
इयं खलु महामुद्रा महासिद्धैः प्रदर्शिता॥ १३॥

(13) Then one should breathe out very slowly without
hurrying up. This has been declared to be Mahāmudrā
by the great siddhas.

महाक्लेशादयो दोषाः क्षीयन्ते मरणादयः।
महामुद्रां च तेनैव वदन्ति विबुधोत्तमाः॥१४॥

(14) The wise great yogīs declare this as Mahāmudrā
and say that through it all the doṣas like great
afflictions of the body, including death, get weakened.

चन्द्राङ्घे   च समभ्यस्य सूर्याङ्घे पुनरभ्यसेत्।
यावत्तुल्या भवेत् सङ्ख्या ततो मुद्रां विसर्जयेत्॥ १५॥

(15) He should first practice on the moon (left side),
and then practice on the sun (right side); when the
number held in both positions becomes equal, then
(the practice of) the Mudrā should be ended (for the
time).

न हि पथ्यमपथ्यं वा रसा: सर्वेऽपि नीरसा:।
अपि भुक्तं विषं घोरं पीयूषमिव जीर्यति॥ १६॥

(16) There is nothing that such a practitioner cannot
eat or must avoid. All food of whatever taste or no
taste at all, and even poison would be thoroughly
digested as if it were nectar.

क्षयकुष्ठगुदावर्त्तगुल्माजीर्णपुरोगमा:।
तस्य दोषा: क्षयं यान्ति महामुद्रां तु योऽभ्यसेत्॥ १७॥

(17) Practice of Mahāmudrā removes consumption,
leprosy, piles, constipation, abdominal diseases,
indigestion etc.

कथितेयं महामुद्रा महासिद्धिकरी नृणाम्।
गोपनीया प्रयत्लेन न देया यस्य कस्यचित्॥ १८॥

(18) Thus has been described the Mahāmudrā that
confers great siddhis on all persons. This should be
carefully kept secret and should not be divulged to any
and every one.

पाणिर्ं वामस्य पादस्य योनिस्थाने नियोजयेत् ।
वामोरूपरि संस्थाप्यं दक्षिणं चरणं तथा ॥ १९ ॥

(19) Mahābandha: Pressing the prineum with the left heel, place the right foot upon the left thigh.

पूरयित्वा ततो वायुं हृदये चिबुकं दृढम् ।
निष्पीड्य योनिमाकुञ्च्य मनोमध्ये नियोजयेत् ॥ २० ॥

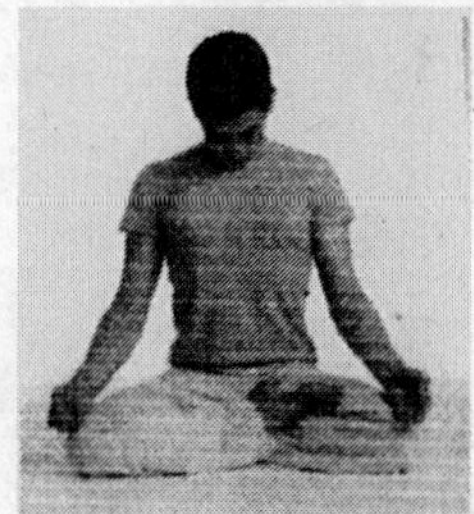

(20) Having drawn in the breath, place the chin firmly on the chest, contract the anus and fix the mind in the middle (on the suṣumnā nāḍī).

धारयित्वा यथाशक्ति रेचयेदनिलं शनैः ।
सव्याङ्गे तु समभ्यस्य दक्षाङ्गे पुनरभ्यसेत् ॥ २१ ॥

(21) Restrain the breath as long as possible, then breathe out slowly. Practice well first on the left side and then on the right side.

मतमत्र तु केषाञ्चित् कण्ठबन्धं विवर्जयेत् ।
राजदन्तस्थजिह्वायां बन्धः शस्तो भवेदिति ॥ २२ ॥

(22) According to some the throat lock (Jālandhara - bandha) should be avoided (here) and the tongue should be pressed firmly against the root of the front teeth.

अयं तु सर्वनाडीनामूर्ध्वगतिनिरोधकः ।
अयं खलु महाबन्धो महासिद्धिप्रदायकः ॥ २३ ॥

(23) This (Jihvā-bandha in the course of the Mahābandha) stops the upward course of the prāṇa through all the nāḍīs, except the suṣumnā. This Mahābandha (helps to) confer great siddhis.

कालपाशमहाबन्धविमोचनविचक्षणः ।
त्रिवेणीसङ्गमं धत्ते केदारं प्रापयेन्मनः ॥ २४ ॥

(24) This frees one from the great noose of Time (death), and brings about the union of the three streams (i.e. nāḍīs : iḍā, piṅgalā and suṣumnā). It also enables the mind to reach Kedāra (the sacred seat of Lord Śiva in the center between the eyebrows).

रूपलावण्यसम्पन्ना यथा स्त्री पुरुषं विना ।
महामुद्रामहाबन्धौ निष्फलौ वेधवर्जिता ॥ २५ ॥

(25) As a beautiful and graceful woman is unfruitful without a husband, so Mahāmudrā and Mahābandha have no value without the Mahāvedha.

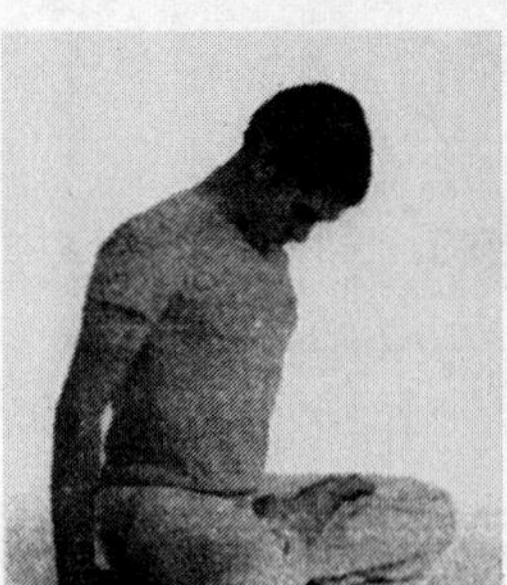

महाबन्धस्थितो योगी कृत्वा पूरकमेकधीः ।
वायूनां गतिमावृत्य निभृतं कण्ठमुद्रया ॥ २६ ॥

(26) Mahāvedha: The yogī, assuming the Mahābandha posture, should draw in his breath with a concentrated mind

and stop the (upward and downward course of the) prāṇa by the throat mudrā (Jālandhara-bandha).

समहस्तयुगो भूमौ स्फिचौ सन्ताडयेच्छनैः ।
पुटद्वयमतिक्रम्य वायुः स्फुरित मध्यगः ॥ २७ ॥

(27) Place the two palms straight upon the ground, and strike (the ground) softly with the buttocks. By this the prāṇa, leaving the two nāḍīs.(iḍā, piṅgalā) goes through the middle (suṣumnā).

सोमसूर्याग्निसम्बन्धो जायते चामृताय वै ।
मृतावस्था समुत्पन्ना ततो वायुं विरेचयेत् ॥ २८ ॥

(28) Then takes place the union of the Moon, Sun and Fire (iḍā, piṅgalā and suṣumnā) that surely leads to immortality. The body then attains a deathlike aspect. Then, breathe out slowly.

महावेधोऽयमभ्यासान्महासिद्धिप्रदायकः ।
वलीपलितवेपघ्नः सेव्यते साधकोत्तमैः ॥ २९ ॥

(29) This is how Mahāvedha is performed. With practice it confers great siddhis, removes wrinkles, gray hairs and trembling. So this is followed by expert practitioners.

एतत्त्रयं महागुह्यं जरामृत्युविनाशनम् ।
वह्निवृद्धिकरं चैव ह्यणिमादिगुणप्रदम् ॥ ३० ॥

(30) These highly esoteric three bandhas ward off death and old age, increase the gastric fire and confer the siddhis such as aṇimā etc.

अष्टधा क्रियते चैव यामे यामे दिने दिने ।
पुण्यसम्भारसन्धायि   पापौघभिदुरं सदा ।
सम्यक् शिक्षावतामेवं स्वल्पं प्रथमसाधनम् ॥ ३१ ॥

(31) These are performed in eight different ways, every day at every yāma (three hours). These bestow puṇya (merit) and destroy the accumulated pāpa (vices). Those who are well tutored in these, after being guided by the teacher, need to practice them gradually.

कपालकुहरे जिह्वा प्रविष्टा विपरीतगा ।
भ्रुवोरन्तर्गता   दृष्टिर्मुद्रा भवति खेचरी ॥ ३२ ॥

(32) Khecarī: The tongue is turned back and enters the cavity leading to the skull and the eyes are fixed firmly between the eyebrows. This is Khecarī mudrā.

छेदनचालनदोहैः   कलां क्रमेण वर्धयेत्तावत् ।
सा यावद् भ्रूमध्यं स्पृशति तदा खेचरीसिद्धिः ॥ ३३ ॥

(33) The Khecarī mudrā becomes successful when the length of the tongue is increased by cutting, shaking and pressing it, until it touches the middle of the eyebrows.

[Not recommended. See Commentary on verse 6.]

स्नुहीपत्रनिभं शस्त्रं सुतीक्ष्णं स्निग्धनिर्मलम् ।
समादाय ततस्तेन रोममात्रं समुच्छिनेत् ॥ ३४ ॥

(34) Taking a smooth, clean knife as sharp as the leaf of the milkhedge plant, cut, to a hair's breadth (the tender membrane that connects the tongue with the lower part of the mouth).

[Not recommended. See Commentary on verse 6.]

तत: सैन्धवपथ्याभ्यां चूर्णिताभ्यां प्रधर्षयेत् ।
पुन: सप्तदिने प्रासे रोममात्रं समुच्छिनेत् ॥ ३५ ॥

(35) Then run the part with a compound of powdered rock salt and harītaki (turmeric). Then after seven days, cut again to the extent of a hair's breadth.

[Not recommended. See Commentary on verse 6.]

एवं क्रमेण षण्मासं नित्यं युक्त:समाचरेत् ।
षण्मासाद्रसनामूलशिराबन्ध: प्रणश्यति ॥ ३६ ॥

(36) Practice gradually and with diligence for a period of six months. In six months the membrane that connects the tongue with the lower part of the mouth is severed.

[Not recommended. See Commentary on verse 6.]

कलां पराङ्मुखीं कृत्वा त्रिपथे परियोजयेत् ।
सा भवेत् खेचरीमुद्रा व्योमचक्रं तदुच्यले ॥ ३७ ॥

(37) Turn the tongue to enter the place at the junction of the three nāḍīs i.e., the hole in the palate. This

Khecarī mudrā is also called Vyomacakra.

रसनामूर्ध्वगां कृत्वा क्षणार्धमपि निष्ठति।
विषैर्विमुच्यते योगी व्याधिमृत्युजरादिभिः ॥ ३८ ॥

(38) When this is kept up even for half a kṣana i.e. for about half an hour with the tongue turned upwards, the body is freed from all poisons, disease, old age and death.

न रोगो मरणं तन्द्रा न निद्रा न क्षुधा तृषा।
न च मूर्च्छा भवेत्तस्य यो मुद्रां वेत्ति खेचरीम्॥ ३९ ॥

(39) One who knows the Khecarī mudrā is free from disease, death, sloth, sleep, hunger, thirst or clouding of the intellect.

पीड्यते न स रोगेण लिप्यते न च कर्मणा।
बाध्यते न स कालेन यो मुद्रां वेत्ति खेचरीम्॥ ४० ॥

(40) He who knows the Khecarī mudrā is not affected by any disease. He is not tainted by any karma, and Time (death) has no power over him.

चित्तं चरति खे यस्माज्जिह्वा चरति खे गता।
तेनैषा   खेचरी नाम मुद्रा सिद्धैर्निरूपिता॥ ४१ ॥

(41) The mudrā is designated as Khecarī by siddhas because the mind moves in space (ākāśa) and the tongue (also) moves in the ākāśa.

खेचर्या मुद्रितं येन विवरं लम्बिकोर्ध्वतः।
न तस्य क्षरते बिन्दुः कामिन्या-श्लेषितस्य च॥ ४२॥

(42) With the cavity at the upper part of the palate sealed through the Khecarī mudrā, the seminal fluid is not emitted even though he is embraced by a passionate woman.

चलितोऽपि यदा बिन्दुः सम्प्राप्तो योनिमण्डलम्।
व्रजत्यूर्ध्वं हतः शक्त्या निबद्धो योनिमुद्रया॥ ४३॥

(43) Even though the fluid has come down to the genital organ, still he can draw it upwards by his powers by practicing yonimudrā.

ऊर्ध्वजिह्वः स्थिरो भूत्वा सोमपानं करोति यः।
मासार्धेन न सन्देहो मृत्युं जयति योगवित्॥ ४४॥

(44) The yogī who with his tongue turned upwards drinks the soma juice with a concentrated mind, undoubtedly conquers death within fifteen days.

[Not recommended. See Commentary on verse 6.]

नित्यं सोमकलापूर्णं शरीरं यस्य योगिनः।
तक्षकेणापि दष्टस्य विषं तस्य न सर्पति॥ ४५॥

(45) When the body of the yogī is filled daily with the soma juice, he does not perish even when bitten by the serpent Takṣaka.

इन्धनानि यथा वह्निस्तैलवर्तिं च दीपक: ।
तथा सोमकलापूर्णं देही देहं न मुञ्चति ॥ ४६ ॥

(46) As the fire does not go out so long as there is fuel, as the light in the lamp does not die out so long as there is oil and wick, so also the jīva (individual self) remains in the body as long as it is vivified by the nectar of the moon.

गोमांसं भक्षयेन्नित्यं पिबेदमरवारूणीम् ।
कुलीनं तमहं मनये चेतरे कुलघातका: ॥ ४७ ॥

(47) One (who is filled with this nectar) may eat the flesh of a cow or drink Amaravāruṇī (strong liquor), but I consider him to be born in the most noble of families, others are destroyers of families.

[Not to be taken literally. See next verse.]

गोशब्देनोदिता जिह्वा तत्प्रवेशो हि तालुनि ।
गोमांसभक्षणं तत्तु महापातकनाशनम् ॥ ४८ ॥

(48) By the word "go" (in Saṁskṛt) is meant the tongue. Making it enter the hole in the palate is "eating the flesh of the go" (cow or the tongue). This destroys the five great pāpas (vices).

जिह्वाप्रवेशसम्भूतवह्निनोत्पादित: खलु ।
चन्द्रात् स्रवति य: सार: स स्यादमरवारूणी ॥ ४९ ॥

*(49) The essence that flows from the moon, which is
produced by the heat caused by the entry of the
tongue, is called Amaravāruṇī.*

चुम्बन्ती यदि लम्बिकाग्रमनिशं जिह्वारसस्यन्दिनी,

सक्षारा कटुकाम्लदुग्धसदृशी मध्वाज्यतुल्या तथा ।

व्याधीनां हरणं जरान्तकरणं शस्त्रागमोदीरणं,

तस्य   स्यादमरत्वमष्टगुणितं सिद्धाङ्गनाकर्षणम् ॥ ५० ॥

*(50) When the tongue touches the cavity in the palate
all the time, the nectar (of the moon) flows; it tastes
salty, pungent and sour, it also resembles milk, honey,
and ghee. This cures all diseases, old age is overcome,
weapons are warded off, immortality is assured, the
eight siddhis come to him and he attracts siddha
women.*

[Not to be taken literally.]

The nectar possesses the tastes of salt, chilli, tamarind, milk, honey,
and ghee, as if it were these things. The tastes vary according to the
times.

मूर्ध्नः षोडशपत्रपद्मगलितं प्राणादवासं हठा-

दूर्ध्वास्यो रसनां नियम्य विवरे शक्तिं परां चिन्तयन् ।

उत्कल्लोलकलाजलं च विमलं धारामयं यः पिबे-

न्निर्व्याधिः स मृणालकोमलवपुर्योगी चिरं जीवति ॥ ५१ ॥

*(51) The yogī with face turned upwards and the hole
in the palate closed firmly by the tongue by
Haṭhayoga, meditates on the Supreme Power
(Kuṇḍalinī, Parāśakti), and drinks the clear stream of*

nectar flowing from the moon into the lotus (in the throat). He is then free of all diseases and has a body soft as a lotus stalk and lives long.

यत्प्रालेयं प्रहितसुषिरं मेरुमूर्धान्तरस्थं
तस्मिंस्तत्त्वं प्रवदति सुधीस्तन्मुखं निम्नगानाम् ।
चन्द्रात्सार: स्रवति वपुषस्तेन मृत्युर्नराणां
तद्बध्नीयात् सुकरणमतो नान्यथा कायसिद्धि: ॥ ५२ ॥

(52) In the interior cavity of the upper part of the Meru (i.e. suśumnā), the fountain head of the nāḍīs, nectar starts flowing. (Performing khecarī mudrā) with pure intellect (full of sattva, devoid of any trace of rajas or tamas), the yogīn sees therein the Ultimate Truth (the Ātman). If the life giving nectar flows uncontrolled, death will result. Therefore, khecarī mudrā should be meticulously practiced to stop this flow downwards and without this the yogīn cannot achieve the perfection of the body.

सुषिरं ज्ञानजनकं पञ्चस्रोत:समन्वितम् ।
तिष्ठते खेचरी मुद्रा तस्मिञ्ज्ञून्ये निरञ्जने ॥ ५३ ॥

(53) The hole is the meeting place of the five nāḍīs bestowing (spiritual) knowledge. Khecarī mudrā stands firm in that pure void.

एकं सृष्टिमयं बीजमेका मुद्रा च खेचरी ।
एको देवो निरालम्ब एकावस्था मनोन्मनी ॥ ५४ ॥

(54) There is only one seed of creation (i.e., OM),
only one mudrā, the Khecarī; only one deity, the one
not dependent on anything; and only one (spiritual)
state i.e. Manonmanī.

बद्धो   येन   सुषुम्नायां प्राणस्तूड्डीयते यतः।
तस्मादुड्डीयनाख्योऽयं योगिभिः समुदाहतः ॥ ५५ ॥

(55) Uḍḍīyānabandha: This bandha is called
Uḍḍīyāna by yogīs by which the prāṇa is arrested and
flies through the suṣumnā.

उड्डीनं कुरुते यस्मादविश्रान्तं महाखगः।
उड्डीयानं   तदेव स्यात्तत्र बन्धोऽभिधीयते॥ ५६ ॥

(56) Because this great bird (prāṇa) flies up
incessantly through suṣumnā, it is called
Uḍḍīyānabandha.

उदरे पश्चिमं तानं नाभेरूर्ध्वं च कारयेत्।
उड्डीयानो ह्यसौ बन्धो मृत्युमातङ्गकेसरी ॥ ५७ ॥

(57) The drawing up of the abdomen above the navel
(so that it rests against the back of the body) is called
uḍḍīyānabandha, and it is like a lion that kills the
elephant "Death".

उड्डीयानं तु सहजं गुरुणा कथितं सदा।
अभ्यसेत्सततं   यस्तु वृद्धोऽपि तरुणायते ॥ ५८ ॥

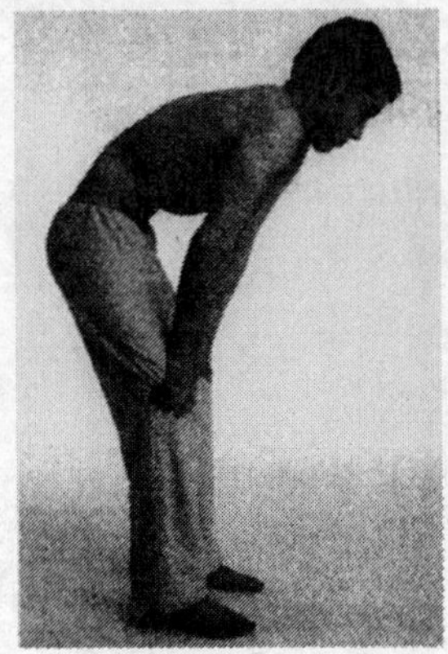

(58) He who constantly practices uddīyānabandha as taught by his guru, so that it becomes natural, becomes young even though he be old.

"Becomes natural" means that it follows naturally after powerful expiration.

नाभेरूर्ध्वमधश्चापि तानं कुर्यात्प्रयत्नतः ।
षण्मासमभ्यसेन्मृत्युं जयत्येव न संशयः ॥ ५९ ॥

(59) He should draw back with effort (the abdomen) above and below the navel, and practice for six months. (Then) without doubt, he conquers death in six months.

सर्वेषामेव   बन्धानामुत्तमो   ह्युड्डियानकः ।
उड्डियाने दृढे बन्धे मुक्तिः स्वाभाविकी भवेत् ॥ ६० ॥

(60) Of all the bandhas, the Uḍḍīyāna is the most excellent. When this has been mastered, mukti (liberation) follows naturally.

पार्णिर्भागेन सम्पीड्य योनिमाकुञ्चयेद्गुदम् ।
अपानमूर्ध्यमाकृष्य   मूलबन्धोऽभिधीयते ॥ ६१ ॥

(61) Mūlabandha: Pressing the perineum with the heel, contract the anus and draw the apāna upwards. This is called mūlabandha.

अधोगतिमपानं वा ऊर्ध्वगं कुरुते बलात् ।
आकुञ्चनेन तं प्राहुर्मूलबन्धं हि योगिन: ॥ ६२ ॥

(62) By contraction of the mūlādhāra, the apāna whose course is downwards, is made to go upwards (through suṣumnā). Therefore the yogīs call it mūlabandha.

गुदं पाष्ण्र्या तु सम्पीड्य वायुमाकुञ्चयेद्बलात् ।
वारं वारं यथा चोर्ध्वं समायाति समीरण: ॥ ६३ ॥

(63) Pressing the anus with the heel, contract the air forcibly and repeatedly until the breath (apāna) goes upwards.

प्राणापानौ नादबिन्दू मूलबन्धेन चैकताम् ।
गत्वा योगस्य संसिद्धिं यच्छतो नात्र संशय: ॥ ६४ ॥

(64) Mūlabandha which unites prāṇa and apāna, nāda and bindu, will doubtless give perfection in Yoga.

अपानप्राणयोरैक्यं क्षयो मूत्रपुरीषयो: ।
युवा भवति वृद्धोऽपि सततं मूलबन्धात् ॥ ६५ ॥

(65) With constant practice, mūlabandha, besides uniting prāṇa and apāna, induces decrease in urine and excrement. Even the aged will become young.

When you properly perform pranayama with bandhas and mudras, along with the right diet, your urination and other excretions become very limited. There is just a little perspiration. This is because there is not much gross poison left in the system.

अपाने ऊर्ध्वगे जाते प्रयाते वह्निमण्डलम् ।
तदाऽनलशिखा दीर्घा जायते वायुनाऽऽहता ॥ ६६ ॥

(66) When the apāna rises upwards and reaches the circle of fire, then the flame of the fire grows long and bright, being fanned by apāna.

This is to be taken symbolically so that you can get a mental picture of how the Kundalini functions. The fire is the Kundalini. Just as the fire becomes bigger when it is fanned by the wind, so when the prana and apana are united, this starts to fan the Kundalini. It becomes brighter.

ततो यातो वह्न्यपानौ प्राणमुष्णस्वरूपकम् ।
तेनात्यन्तप्रदीप्तस्तु ज्वलनो देहजस्तथा ॥ ६७ ॥

(67) When the apāna and the fire join prāṇa, which is naturally hot, then the heat in the body becomes considerably bright and intensified.

This is not physical heat; it is psychic heat, and you can see the radiations. It is said that a true yogi's body will shine even in advanced age. There will be no wrinkles.

तेन कुण्डलिनी सुप्ता सन्तप्ता सम्प्रबुध्यते ।
दण्डाहता भुजङ्गीव निश्वस्य ऋजुतां व्रजेत् ॥ ६८ ॥

(68) As a result, Kuṇḍalinī which is asleep, feeling the extreme heat awakens, just as a serpent struck by a stick hisses and straightens itself.

Again, this symbolizes awakening of the Kundalini. Of course there is no serpent there. The energy which is dormant (static), becomes kinetic (or dynamic).

बिलं प्रविष्टेव ततो ब्रह्मनाड्यन्तरं व्रजेत् ।
तस्मान्नित्यं मूलबन्ध: कर्त्तव्यो योगिभि: सदा ॥ ६९ ॥

(69) Then it (Kuṇḍalinī) goes into its hole, i.e., the interior of brahmanāḍī. Therefore, the yogīs should always practice mūlabandha.

"Always" means that you concentrate. Breathing from the bottom, feel that the Kundalini is going up, all the while repeating your mantra.

कण्डमाकुञ्चय हृदये स्थापयेच्चिबुकं दृढम् ।
बन्धो जालन्धराख्योऽयं जरामृत्युविनाशक: ॥ ७० ॥

(70) Jālandharabandha: Contract the throat and depress the chin firmly against the chest. This is jālandhara-bandha. It destroys old age and death.

बध्नाति हि सिराजालमधोगामि नभोजलम् ।
ततो जालन्धरो बन्ध: कण्ठदु:खौघनाशन: ॥ ७१ ॥

(71) It is called jālandhara-bandha because it tightens the network of nāḍīs and stops the downward flow of the nectar (from the throat). This bandha destroys the illnesses of the throat.

जालन्धरे कृते बन्धे कण्ठसङ्कोचलक्षणे ।
न पीयूषं पतत्यग्नौ न च वायु: प्रकुप्यति ॥ ७२ ॥

(72) In this bandha, due to the contraction at the throat, no drop of the nectar falls into the gastric fire

and prāṇa does not go in the wrong way,
(i.e., in the space between the nāḍīs).

कण्ठसङ्कोचनेनैव द्वे नाड्यो स्तम्भयेद् दृढम्।
मध्यचक्रमिदं   ज्ञेयं   षोडशाधारबन्धनम्॥ ७३ ॥

(73) By the firm contraction of the throat, the two
nāḍīs are fixed. Here in the throat is situated the
middle cakra, the viśuddhi. This binds firmly the
sixteen ādhāras or vital centres.

मूलस्थानं समाकुञ्च्य उड्डियानं तु कारयेत्।
इडां च पिङ्गलां बध्वा वाहयेत् पश्चिमे पथि॥ ७४॥

(74) Contracting the anus, practice the
uḍḍīyānabandha. Tighten firmly the iḍā and piṅgalā
(jālandhara-bandha), and cause the breath to flow
through the upper path, i.e., suṣumnā.

अनेनैव   विधानेन प्रयाति पवनो लयम्।
ततो न जायते मृत्युर्जरारोगादिकं तथा॥ ७५ ॥

(75) By this method the breath becomes steady
(remains motionless in the suṣumnā). Then there is no
disease, old age or death.

बन्धत्रयमिदं श्रेष्ठं महासिद्धैश्च सेवितम्।
सर्वेषां हठतन्त्राणां साधनं योगिनो विदुः॥ ७६ ॥

(76) These three fold excellent bandhas are practiced by the great siddhas. The yogīs know that the practice of these ensures success in the Haṭhayoga practices.

यत्किञ्चित् स्रवते चन्द्रादमृतं दिव्यरूपिण: ।
तत्सर्वं ग्रसते सूर्यस्तेन पिण्डो जरायुत: ॥ ७७ ॥

(77) Every particle of nectar that flows from the ambrosial Moon is swallowed up by the Sun. Hence the body becomes old.

According to the Yoga system, we get old because the ambrosial energy coming from the higher centers is swallowed by the Sun. It is just like water dripping into a fire. Every day, from consuming this energy, eventually old age results. But if you reverse this process by stopping the flow for a certain time, then the Sun won't swallow the energy. There is no way that I can explain this properly in scientific terms because we are not talking about physical energy, but about astral or psychic waves. The "all-consuming Sun" is the fire center at the navel. We stop this flow with the practice of Viparita karani as described below.

तत्रास्ति करणं दिव्यं सूर्यस्य मुखञ्चनम् ।
गुरूपदेशतो ज्ञेयं न तु शस्त्रार्थकोटिभि: ॥ ७८ ॥

(78) There is a most excellent process by which the Sun is deceived. This should be learned from the guru himself. A theoretical study of crores of śāstras cannot throw any light upon it.

Here they are giving you a warning. It is not a mere physical process which is being described below, but it is the movement of psychic energy (prana and apana). Moreover, it is not the physical Sun and the physical Moon which was referred to above; they are psychic phenomena. Words cannot explain these things so you must learn from a guru.

ऊर्ध्वं नाभेरधस्तालोरूर्ध्वं भानुरध: शशी ।
करणी विपरीताख्या गुरुवाक्येन लभ्यते ॥ ७९ ॥

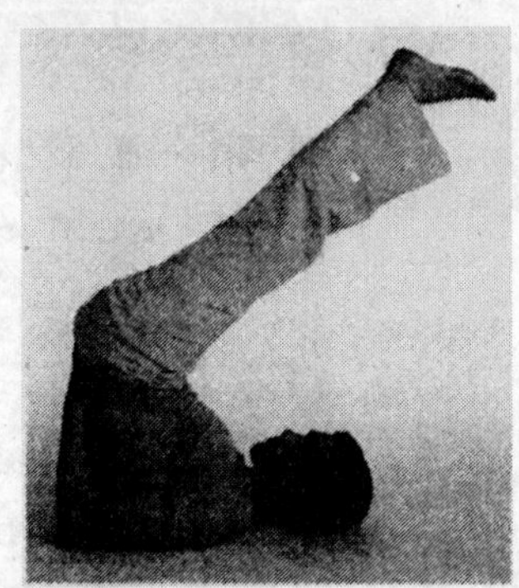

*(79) Sun and Moon assume
exactly reverse positions, i.e.
Sun that is now below the
navel, and the Moon that is
above the palate, change
plate. This is learnt from the
guru.*

नित्यमभ्यासयुक्तस्य   जठराग्निविवर्धिनी ।
आहरो बहुलस्तस्य सम्पाद्य: साधकस्य च ॥ ८० ॥

*(80) In the case of one who practices this daily, the
gastric fire is increased. Therefore, the yogī should
always have a large quantity of food ready.*

That you all don't mind at all, I know. Actually, this should be
understood to mean nutritious food.

अल्पाहारो यदि भवेदग्निर्दहति   तत्क्षणात् ।
अध: शिराश्चोर्ध्वपाद: क्षणं स्यात् प्रथमे दिने ॥ ८१ ॥

*(81) If he stints on his diet, the fire consumes the
body.*

This means that you should not fast while following intensive
practice.

*On the first day, he should stand for a moment upon
his head, with his heels in the air.*

This differs from the shoulderstand, since in the shoulderstand the pressure is on the Vishudha chakra as well as on the thyroid and parathyroid glands. Here, as there is no pressure on those places the pranic energy flows.

क्षणाच्च किञ्चिदधिकमभ्यसेच्च दिने दिने।
वलितं पलितं चैव षण्मासोर्ध्वं न दृश्यते।
याममात्रं तु यो नित्यमभ्यसेत् स तु कालजित्॥८२॥

(82) While practicing this, increase the duration gradually every day. After six months of regular practice wrinkles and grey hair disappear. He who practices this for a yāma i.e., three hours daily, conquers death.

स्वेच्छया वर्तमानोऽपि योगोक्तैर्नियमैर्विना।
वज्रोलीं यो विजानाति स योगी सिद्धिभाजनम्॥८३॥

(83) Vajrolīmudrā: Even though living an ordinary life without observing the yoga regulations, still if one practices the vajrolīmudrā, that person becomes possessed of the siddhis.

(84 - 103) These verses have been omitted, as they describe Vajrolī, Sahajolī, and Amarolī mudrās, which are not followed in sāttvic sādhana.

कुटिलाङ्गी कुण्डलिनी भुजङ्गी शक्तिरीश्वरी।
कुण्डल्यरुन्धती चैते शब्दा: पर्यायवाचका:॥१०४॥

(104) *Śakticālana: Kuṭilāṅgī, kuṇḍalinī Bhujaṅgī, Śakti, Īṣvarī, and Arundhatī are synonymous (or Kuṇḍalinī).*

उद्घाटयेत्कपाटं तु यथा कुञ्चिकया हठात्।
कुण्डलिन्या तथा योगी मोक्षद्वारं विभेदयेत्॥ १०५ ॥

(105) *As one forces open a door with a key, so the yogī should force open the door to mokṣa by the power of Kuṇḍalinī.*

येन मार्गेण गन्तव्यं ब्रह्मस्थानं निरामयम्।
मुखेनाच्छाद्य तद्द्वारं प्रसुप्ता परमेश्वरी॥ १०६ ॥

(106) *Parameśvari (the primeval, Great Goddess) sleeps closing with her mouth the hole through which one should go to the Brahmarandhra (the seat of Brahman), where there is no pain or misery.*

कन्दोर्ध्वे कुण्डलीशक्तिः सुप्ता मोक्षाय योगिनाम्।
बन्धनाय च मूढानां यस्तां वेत्ति स योगवित्॥ १०७ ॥

(107) *That Kuṇḍalinī Śakti, which the yogīs know, sleeps above the kanda (the place near the navel where the nāḍīs unite and separate). It gives mukti to the yogīs and bondage to the fools. He who knows her, knows Yoga.*

When the Kundalini is dormant, in a low vibratory state, you only understand sensual and sexual life. But when it is in a subtle state it gives liberation.

He knows the Shakti which is hidden in all of us.

कुण्डली कुटिलाकारा   सर्पवत्परिकीर्त्तिता।
सा शक्तिश्चलिता येन से मुक्तो नात्र संशय: ॥१०८॥

(108) Kuṇḍalinī is described as being coiled like a serpent. He who causes that Śakti to move (from the Mūlādhāra upwards) becomes free, without doubt.

गङ्गायमुनयोर्मध्ये   बालरण्डां तपस्विनीम्।
बलात्कारेण गृह्णीयात्तद्विष्णो: परमं पदम्॥१०९॥

(109) Between the Gaṅgā and the Yamumā, there sits the young widow, practicing austerity. She should be seized by force. That leads to the supreme seat of Viṣṇu.

If you are a yogi, you must be able to correctly interpret such things. See next verse.

इडा भगवती   गङ्गा पिङ्गला यमुना नदी।
इडापिङ्गलयोर्मध्ये बालरण्डा च कुण्डली॥११०॥

(110) Iḍā is the sacred Gaṅgā, piṅgalā is the river Yamunā. Between iḍā and piṅgalā there sits the young widow Kuṇḍalinī.

Why is the Kundalini Shakti called "widow" here? It is because she is not with Siva. Siva is in the Sahasrara, so she is alone, a widow. Simple language is used, but it is all very difficult for Westerners to understand on their own.

पुच्छे   प्रगृह्य भुजगीं सुषामामुद्बोधयेच्च ताम्।
निद्रां विहाय सा शक्तिरूर्ध्वमुत्तिष्ठते हठात्॥१११॥

(111) You should awaken the sleeping serpent by taking hold of its tail. The Śakti leaving off sleep, goes up with force by Haṭhayoga.

How do you take hold and shake its tail? By bandhas and mudras.

अवस्थिता चैव फणावती सा प्रातश्च सायं प्रहरार्धमात्रम् ।
प्रपूर्य सूर्यात् परिधानयुक्त्या प्रगृह्य नित्यं परिचालनीया ॥ ११२ ॥

(112) Having inhaled through the right nostril (piṅgalā), the recumbent serpent should be taken hold of by the process of paridhāna, and made to move daily for an hour and a half, both morning and evening.

This refers to Alternate Nostril Breathing, Surya bheda, and other pranayamas.

Then he should manipulate this Shakti for about an hour and a half at both morning and evening twilights.

You must shake the "tail" for an hour and a half.

Note: see The Serpent Power, 1964, p. 207.

ऊर्ध्वं वितस्तिमात्रं तु विस्तारं चतुरङ्गुलम् ।
मृदुलं धवलं प्राक्तं वेष्टिताम्बरलक्षणम् ॥ ११३ ॥

(113) (The kanda) is twelve inches above the anus and four inches both ways in extension. It has been described as soft and white as if covered with a cloth.

It is the approximate area where all the plexuses are joined together at the Muladhara. This is where the energy is dormant.

It is soft and white because in the spinal cord there is also white matter. This was written thousands of years ago.

This is because their spinal cords are quite different. [From the kanda spring the 72,000 nadis.] This is like a battery, with wires going to numerous areas. This is why, when the nadis are not purified properly by bandhas and pranayama, etc., the prana goes through wrong nadis and you get psychological problems.

सति वज्रासने पादौ कराभ्यां धारयेद् दृढम् ।
गुल्फदेशसमीपे च कन्दं तत्र प्रपीडयेत्॥ ११४ ॥

(114) Seated in the Vajrāsana posture, firmly take hold of the feet near the ankles and thereby put pressure on the kanda.

This is really what we call Siddhasana; sometimes it was called Vijrasana by different teachers. This is because "Vajrasana" literally means "energy asana," so it was applied to any asana which was used for the raising of the energy. Vajra was the thunderbolt weapon of Indra.

वज्रासने स्थितो योगी चालयित्वा च कुण्डलीम् ।
कुर्यादनन्तरं भस्त्रां कुण्डलीमाशु बोधयेत्॥ ११५ ॥

(115) Having thus caused Kuṇḍalinī to move after assuming Vajrāsana, perform Bhastrikā kumbhaka; this should soon awaken Kuṇḍalinī.

This is Shakti chalani.

भानोराकुञ्चनं कुर्यात् कुण्डलीं चालयेत् ततः ।
मृत्युवक्त्रगतस्यापि तस्य मृत्युभयं कुतः ॥ ११६ ॥

(116) He should then contract the Sun (near the navel) and then cause the Kuṇḍalinī to move. Even though he is in the mouth of death, where can there be any fear of death for such a one?

What is meant by "contract the sun?" Uddiyana bandha. This is an extremely advanced practice, after years of training. It is not necessary to go too deeply into this subject here. If this is practiced early there will be no results because of the existence of blocks and impurities in the Sushumna.

मुहूर्त्तद्वयपर्यन्तं   निर्भयं   चालनादसौ।
ऊर्ध्वमाकृष्यते किञ्चित् सुषुम्नायां समुद्गता॥ ११७॥

(117) When Kuṇḍalinī is moved fearlessly for two muhūrtas, she who has entered the suṣumnā is drawn (upwards) a little more.

Waves of energy start moving, slowly, slowly upwards.

तेन   कुण्डलिनी तस्याः सुषुम्राया मुखं ध्रुवम्।
जहाति तस्मात् प्राणोऽयं सुषुम्नां व्रजति स्वतः॥ ११८॥

(118) By this Kuṇḍalinī certainly leaves (open) the mouth of the suṣumnā, and the prāna goes naturally to suṣumnā.

तस्मात् सञ्चालयेन्नित्यं सुखसुप्तामरुन्धतीम्।
तस्याः संचालनेनैव योगी रोगैः प्रमुच्यते॥ ११९॥

(119) So, one should move daily the Arundhatī (Kuṇḍalinī) that is calmly sleeping. By moving her, the yogī is freed from diseases.

येन सञ्चालिता शक्ति: स योगी सिद्धिभाजनम्।
किमत्र बहुनोक्तेन कालं जयति लीलया॥ १२० ॥

(120) That yogī by whom Śakti is moved is blessed with all the siddhis. What is the use of speaking so much? He playfully conquers Time (death).

Mere speaking is not sufficient, you must practice.

ब्रह्मचर्यरतस्यैव   नित्यं   हितमिताशिन:।
मण्डलाद् दृश्यते सिद्धि: कुण्डल्यभ्यासयोगिन: ॥ १२१ ॥

(121) Only a yogī who is celibate, who consumes a moderate and nutritious diet and who constantly practices (the awakening of the Kuṇḍalinī) attains perfection within forty days.

This is possible only if many of your impurities have been removed in past incarnations. Then, a bit of practice and perhaps an "OM" from the guru, might be sufficient for this to take place. But if it doesn't happen, you just keep practicing your sadhana until you find success in your next life or in your tenth life from now. Sometimes your old karma may come and create all kinds of obstacles such as sicknesses, etc. Sometimes the karma burns very slowly. When you start intense sadhana, then things may become very intense for you. You may think that you are getting worse, but actually you are burning your karma very quickly in a very short time. Whenever I go into seclusion, most of my karma comes up to be burnt out. I developed frostbite, an accident to my knee, and other things.

कुण्डलीं चालयित्वा तु भस्त्रां कुर्याद्द्विशेषतः।
एवमभ्यस्यतो नित्यं यमिनो यमभीः कुतः॥१२२॥

(122) Having moved the Kuṇḍalini, he should practice in particular the Bhastrikā-kumbhaka. Where can there be the fear of death from Yama for the yogī who practices in this manner constantly?

द्वासप्ततिसहस्राणां नाडीनां मलशोधने।
कुतः प्रक्षालनोपायः कुण्डल्यभ्यसनादृते॥ १२३॥

(123) Besides the practice of Kuṇḍalini, what other means is there for clearing away the impurities of the 72,000 nāḍīs?

इयं तु मध्यमा नाडी दृढाभ्यासेन योगिनाम्।
आसनप्राणसंयाममुद्राभिः सरला भवेत्॥ १२४॥

(124) By persevering in the practice along with āsanas, prāṇayāma and mudrās, the middle nāḍī (suṣumnā) becomes straight.

अभ्यासे तु विनिद्राणां मनोधृत्वा समाधिना।
रुद्राणी वा परा मुद्रा भद्रां सिद्धिं प्रयच्छति॥ १२५॥

(125) With firm concentration of the mind he who practises samādhi without sleep (being alert), he acquires various siddhis conferred by rudrāṇī or by such superior mudrās.

राजयोगं बिना पृथ्वी राजयोगं विना निशा।
राजयोगं विना मुद्रा विचित्रापि न शोभते॥ १२६॥

(126) There is no prithvī (firmness in āsanas)
without Rājayoga. There is no night (kumbhaka)
without the Rājayoga. The various mudrās become
useless without Rājayoga.

मारुतस्य विधिं सर्वं मनोयुक्तं समभ्यसेत्।
इतरत्र न कर्त्तव्या मनोवृत्तिर्मनीषिणा॥ १२७॥

(127) All the processes with regard to the breath
(prāṇa) should be gone through with a mind
concentrated on it. The wise man should not allow his
mind to wander away during that time.

इति मुद्रा दश प्रोक्ता आदिनाथेन शम्भुना।
एकैका तासु यमिनां महासिद्धिप्रदायिनी॥ १२८॥

(128) Thus have the ten mudrās been described by
Ādinātha. By any one of these, one possessed of self-
restraint might obtain great siddhis.

उपदेशं हि मुद्राणां यो दत्ते साम्प्रदायिकम्।
स एव श्रीगुरुः स्वामी साक्षादीश्वर एव सः॥ १२९॥

(129) He who teaches the secret of these mudrās as
handed down by tradition is the real guru, and can be
called Īṣvara in human form.

तस्य वाक्यपरो भूत्वा मुद्राभ्यासे समाहितः ।
अणिमादिगुणैः सार्धं लभते कालवञ्चनम् ॥ १३० ॥

इति श्रीस्वात्मारामयोगीन्द्रविरचितायां
हठयोगप्रदीपिकायां मुद्राविधानं नाम तृतीयोपदेशः ॥

(130) The person following carefully the words of the guru, and attentively practicing the mudrās, obtains the siddhis: aṇimā, etc., as also the art of deceiving death.

Thus ends the third chapter (upadeśa) of *Haṭha Yoga Pradīpīkā* written by Svātmārāma, best of yogīs, called the mudrāvidhāna.

हठयोगप्रदीपिका
Haṭha Yoga Pradīpīkā
CHAPTER FOUR

नमः शिवाय गुरवे नादबिन्दुकलात्मने ।
निरञ्जनपदं याति नित्यं यत्र परायणः ॥ १ ॥

(1) Salutations to Lord Śiva, the divine guru, who is of the form of nāda, bindu and kalā. The person ever-devoted to these, obtains the stainless state (free from Māyā).

नमः शिवाय गुरवे नादबिन्दुकलात्मने।
निरञ्जनपदं याति नित्यं यत्र परायणः ॥ १ ॥

*(1) Salutations to Lord Śiva, the divine guru, who is
of the form of nāda, bindu and kalā. The person ever-
devoted to these, obtains the stainless state (free from
Māyā).*

Nada means sound or wave energy. Bindu means dot; here the dot
is the center or the nucleus. Kala means that which is the
transcendental wave; it ends with a timeless state, a spaceless state,
a non-dual state. Nada and bindu are like Siva and Shakti. Bindu
is like the nucleus in an atom, nada is the electrons whirling
around the nucleus, and the energy is kala. When the nada and
bindu are changed into its wavelength, it becomes energy: a pure
wave. Lord Siva has condensed everything; nada (the sound
energy), bindu (the static force), and kala (the transcendental
energy).

अथेदानीं   प्रवक्ष्यामि समाधिक्रममुत्तमम्।
मृत्युघ्नं च सुखोपायं ब्रह्मानन्दकरं परम् ॥ २ ॥

*(2) Now I shall expound the excellent process of
samādhi that destroys death, and which is the means
to attain great happiness of Brahmānanda (the bliss
of Brahman).*

In [Raja] Yoga there are eight steps. We have been considering
asanas, pranayama, dharana, dhyana, etc., and now we come to
samadhi, the final stage. According to Hatha Yoga, these eight
steps are nothing but progression in pranayama. This means that
when the prana stays in the Sushumna for a certain time, it is called
pratyahara; when it stays a little longer, it is called dharana
(concentration); even longer, it is called dhyana (meditation); and
for an even longer period, it is called samadhi. Samadhi is said to
destroy death because you now understand that you are not the

body but the Immortal Self. Our goal is this Ananda or Bliss. The Supreme Bliss of being absorbed in Brahman is Sat-Chit-Ananda (Existence-Knowledge-Bliss Absolute), or God. Just as a drop of water merges with the ocean and becomes the ocean itself, so the individual merges with the Supreme.

राजयोग: समाधिश्च उन्मनी च मनोन्मनी।
अमरत्वं लयस्तत्त्वं शून्याशून्यं परं पदम्॥ ३ ॥

अमनस्कं तथाद्वैतं निरालम्बं निरञ्जनम्।
जीवन्मुक्तिश्च सहजा तुर्या चेत्येकवाचका: ॥ ४ ॥

(3-4) Rājyoga, samādhi, Unmanī, Manonmanī, Amaratva (immortality), Laya (absorption), Tattva, Śūnyāṣūnya (void and yet non-void), Paramapada, Amanaska (suspended operation of the mind), Advaita (non-dualism), Nirālamba (without support), Nirañjana (pure), Jīvanmukti (liberation while still living), Sahajā (natural state), and Turīya (the fourth state) - are all synonyms.

Samadhi has various names, and these are the names. Raja Yoga is when the mind is still, without any waves. Samadhi is when the mind doesn't function any more and you see your Self (Atman) clearly, or when there is Oneness with Brahman. Unmani is Hatha Yoga samadhi; it refers to the state in which the prana and apana are united and go the higher chakras. Manomani literally means "that which brings joy to the mind," and the only thing which brings joy is the Self, the Atman. Immortality refers to transcending the body so that you identify with the Atman. Concentration is on the Atman: "I am that Brahman." Shunyashunya means void and not void because in that state there is no time, space or causation, but yet one feels pure consciousness and awareness, extreme bliss and happiness. Paramapada means the highest state. Amanaska comes from "manas," meaning mind, and "a" meaning not. When there is not mind, there is no time, space nor causation. Advaita, the non-dual state, is also called Asamprajnata samadhi. In the Niralamba state Atman or Brahman has no support, it is everywhere, it supports everything. Niranjana is pure Consciousness. Jivanmukti is the liberated state. Sahajavastha is the natural state: Sat-Chit-Ananda. Turiya is the superconscious state. All of these terms refer to the same thing.

सलिले सैन्धवं यद्वत्साम्यं भजति योगतः ।
तथात्ममनसोरैक्यं   समाधिरभिधीयते ॥ ५ ॥

(5) Salt in water unites and becomes one with it, so also the identity of Ātman and the mind is known as samādhi.

Here again is another definition of samadhi. When salt is thrown into water, it becomes one with the water. In the same way, the mind and the soul are united so that at that time there is only oneness, or samadhi.

यदा सङ्क्षीयते प्राणो मानसं च प्रलीयते ।
तदा समरसत्वं च समाधिरभिधीयते ॥ ६ ॥

(6) When the prāṇa is without any movement and the mind is absorbed in the Self, then there is a state of harmony; this is known as samādhi.

That prana which creates the inhalation and exhalation, and the apana which goes to the sexual organs and which creates thoughts, are stopped, then the state which remains is your Self: "I Am." This also is called samadhi.

तत्समं च द्वयोरैक्यं जीवात्मपरमात्मनोः ।
प्रनष्टसर्वसङ्कल्पः समाधिः सोऽभिधीयते ॥ ७ ॥

(7) The identity of Jīvātman and Paramātman, and a state of harmony in which there is the cessation of all thoughts, is known as samādhi.

The Jivatman is the individual soul. It unites with the Supreme Brahman or Pramatman or God. When this union takes place, then we can truly say that "I and my Father are one." I is the individual; Father is the Supreme. That union is called samadhi.

राजयोगस्य माहात्म्यं को वा जानाति तत्त्वतः।
ज्ञानं मुक्तिः स्थितिः सिद्धिर्गुरुवाक्येन लभ्यते॥८॥

(8) Who indeed really knows the greatness of Rājayoga in truth? Perfections (like) jñāna, mukti, sthiti and siddhis are obtained only through the instructions of the guru.

When Raja yogis achieve full control over the mind, then they reach the Immortal State. Jnana is the direct cognition of one's own Atman as Parabrahman, mukti is vedeha mukti, sthiti is jivanmukti, and siddhis are anima, etc.

दुर्लभो विषयत्यागो दुर्लभं तत्त्वदर्शनम्।
दुर्लभा सहजावस्था सद्गुरोः करुणां विना॥९॥

(9) Without the compassion of the right guru, abandonment of (attachment to) sense objects is difficult; it is difficult to obtain the insight to truth and the sahajāvasthā (true natural state) is difficult to obtain.

For the guru's grace one should have devotion. Without devotion, your own efforts in pranayama, etc. will not bring success because of the many obstacles. So the grace of God and of guru is very essential.

Indifference to worldly pleasures is vairagya (dispassion). This world is nothing but a mirage. As there is no true happiness, you want to find the eternal happiness which is within you (you are that happiness). Until you have that dispassion, you will not be able to put full effort behind your Yoga practice, so that eventually your vairagya will dissipate, causing you to go back into your old ruts: drinking, smoking, etc. Therefore, you must truly realize that all this drinking and smoking will bring you pain and disease, and you must wish to escape from this. If you realize that you will have to be reincarnated to come back again and again to go through the same learning experiences, you will want to get out of this cycle. Then you will take Yoga seriously and you will have the energy to do this work.

विविधैरासनैः कुम्भैर्विचित्रैः करणैरपि।
प्रबुद्धायां महाशक्तौ प्राणः शून्ये प्रलीयते ॥ १० ॥

(10) When the great power (Kuṇḍalinī) has been roused by the various āsanas, kumbhakas and mudrās, the prāṇa lies hidden in the void (Brahmarandhra).

Through asanas you are regulating the prana. Asanas divert the prana from one area to another, increase or reduce the vibratory level or charge specific areas. Asanas which apply pressure on the solar plexus increase the vibratory level. The lumbar region (lower back) is where the Kundalini Shakti resides. When we loosen those vertebrae so that the discs are no longer compressed, we reduce pressure on the physical nerves, and this in turn affects the astral nerves. Asanas are not just physical exercise. The purpose of all asanas is to reduce this blocked energy. Together with pranayama, bandhas, and mudras, you try to awaken the Kundalini, and when the prana goes in the Sushumna, this state is called Shunya, or vacuum. It is not a physical vacuum; it means that there is no time or space awareness.

उत्पन्नशक्तिबोधस्य तयक्तनिःशेषकर्मण।
योगिनः सहजावस्था स्वयमेव प्रजायते ॥ ११ ॥

(11) Of the yogī in whom the (Kuṇḍḍalinī) Śakti is awakened and who is free of all karmas, the truly natural state of samādhi comes into being on its own.

The purpose is not to force anything; it is a natural process. From watering the plant, eventually you will get flowers and fruits. In the same way, from asanas, pranayama, japa, etc., practiced regularly and increased little by little, the Kundalini automatically awakens. There is no fast or easy method; each individual has to find his own evolutionary rate. Each river has its own level beyond which it will overflow, or if its flow is too low, it will dry out before it reaches the ocean. In the same way, you have to practice regularly and avoid too much enthusiasm in the beginning. Try to find the middle path, then eventually you will reach that state.

सुषुम्नावाहिनि प्राणे शून्ये विशति मानसे।
तदा सर्वाणि कर्माणि निर्मूलयति योगवित्॥ १२ ॥

(12) When the prāṇa moves in the suṣumnā and the mind is absorbed in the Śūnya (void), the intelligent yogī (he who can end the modifications of the mind) uproots all karma.

अमराय नमस्तुभ्यं सोऽपि कालस्त्वया जितः।
पतितं वदने यस्य जगदेतच्चराचरम्॥ १३ ॥

(13) Salutations to you the immortal one, by whom time (death) has been conquered, and into whose mouth all movable and immovable (beings) of the universe fall.

Svatmarama calls those yogis who have conquered time by bringing the Kundalini Shakti into the Sushumna, "Amaras," immortals. You are all immortal, but it is necessary to acquire that knowledge that you are no longer bound by time, space, causation, birth, death, change. This is the author's benediction, not to the body, but to the Higher Self, now realized.

चित्ते समत्वमापन्ने वायौ व्रजति मध्यमे।
तदाऽमरोली वज्रोली सहजोली प्रजायते॥ १४॥

(14) When the mind has reached a state of equanimity and the prāṇa moves through the suṣumnā, then one obtains Amarolī, Vajrolī and Sahajolī.

In time, the various mudras and bandhas come automatically.

ज्ञानं कुतो मनसि सम्भवतीह तावत्
   प्राणोऽपि जीवति मनो म्रियते न यावत्।
प्राणो मनो द्वयमिदं विलयं नयेद्यो
   मोक्षं स गच्छति नरो न कथञ्चिदन्यः॥ १५॥

(15) When the prāṇa lives (is active) and the mind is not dead, till such time, how can jñāna (spiritual knowledge) arise in the mind? He who causes both prāṇa and mind to become quiet obtains mokṣa. No other person can do so.

Jnana is knowledge of the Atman (Self, or God). You cannot obtain God Realization or Self Realization unless prana is brought into the Sushumna. When only the Ida and Pingala are functioning, it is impossible to reach this state. Stopping the Ida and Pingala, and getting the prana into the Sushumna is the purpose of all Yogas. Without that you have knowledge only of the body and you identify with it. That is what the author means by saying "his prana lives." This state is called ajnana (non-knowledge); it is ignorance, "I am the body" is ignorance: "I am the Atman" is Knowledge.

When the prana and apana are withdrawn from the left and right sides and enter into the Sushumna, then the mind becomes extinct. This means that the mind is no longer operating in the ordinary sense. According to Hatha Yoga, moksha is obtained only by those people who are able to practice this.

ज्ञात्वा सुषुम्नासद्भेदं कृत्वा वायुं च मध्यगम् ।
स्थित्वा   सदैव सुस्थाने ब्रह्मरन्ध्रे निरोधयेत् ॥ १६ ॥

(16) Having known the secret of finding the way into the suṣumnā and forcing the prāṇa into it, the yogī should then, seating himself in a convenient spot, restrain his prāṇa in the Brahmarandhra.

सूर्याचन्द्रमसौ धत्तः कालं रात्रिंदिवात्मकम् ।
भौक्त्री   सुषुम्ना कालस्य गुह्यमेतदुदाहृतम् ॥ १७ ॥

(17) The sun and moon are said to regulate day and night. Suṣumnā is said to swallow time. This secret has been explained.

द्वासप्ततिसहस्त्राणि   नाडीद्वाराणि   पञ्जरे ।
सुषुम्ना शाम्भवी शक्तिः शेषास्त्वेव निरर्थकाः ॥ १८ ॥

(18) There are 72,000 nāḍīs in this body. Suṣumnā is the middle nāḍī, containing the Sāmbhavī Śakti. The others (iḍā, piṅgalā etc.) are not of much use.

वायुः परिचितो यस्मादग्निना सह कुण्डलीम् ।
बोधयित्वा   सुषुम्नायां   प्रविशेदनिरोधतः ॥ १९ ॥

(19) With vāyu controlled, the Kuṇḍalinī is aroused along with jaṭharāgni. Then it should be made to enter (suṣumnā) with ease..

सुषुम्नावाहिनि प्राणे सिद्ध्यत्येव मनोन्मनी ।
अन्यथात्वितराभ्यासाः प्रयासायैव योगिनाम् ॥ २० ॥

(20) The prāṇa must flow through the suṣumnā to reach up the Manonmanā state. If not, other practices are only useless efforts.

पवनो बध्यते येन मनस्तेनैव बध्यते ।
मनश्च बध्यते येन पवनस्तेन बध्यते ॥ २१ ॥

(21) He who suspends (restrains) the breath, also restrains the mind. He who has controlled the mind, also controls the breath.

हेतुहयं तु चित्तस्य वासना च समीरणः ।
तयोर्विनष्ट एकस्मिंस्तौ द्वावपि विनश्यतः ॥ २२ ॥

(22) Prāṇa and vāsanas (acquired tendencies/ impressions) activate the mind. When one of these ceases, the other also ceases.

मनो यत्र विलीयेत पवनस्तत्र लीयते ।
पवनो लीयते यत्र मनस्तत्र विलीयते ॥ २३ ॥

(23) Where the mind is quietened, there the prāṇa is absorbed; and where the prāṇa is absorbed, there the mind is quietened.

दुग्धाम्बुवत् सम्मिलितावुभौ तौ तुल्यक्रियौ मानसमारुतौ हि।
यतो मरुतत्र मनः प्रवृत्तिर्यतो मनस्तत्र मरुत्प्रवत्तिः॥ २४॥

(24) Like milk and water mind and prāṇa have affinity for each other and are mingled, and they have similar activities. Where prāṇa goes, there the mind is active; where mind goes, there the prāṇa is active.

तत्रैकनाशादपरस्य नाश एकप्रवृत्तेरपरप्रवृत्तिः।
अध्वस्तयोश्चेन्द्रियवर्गवृत्तिः प्रध्वस्तयोर्मोक्षपदस्य सिद्धिः॥ २५॥

(25) If one is destroyed, the other is also destroyed. If one is active, the other is also active. When they are not destroyed, all the indriyas (the senses) are active. When the two are restrained, mokṣa is attained.

रसस्य मनसश्चैव चञ्चलत्वं स्वभावतः।
रसो बद्धो मनो बद्धं किं न सिद्ध्यति भूतले॥ २६॥

(26) Mind and mercury are unsteady by nature. When mercury is controlled, mind is restrained. What is not possible on the face of this earth?

मूर्च्छितो हरते व्याधीन् मृतो जीवयति स्वयम्।
बद्धः खेचरतां धत्ते रसो वायुश्च पार्वति॥ २७॥

(27) O Pārvati! Mercury and prāṇa when restrained destroy all diseases; when they are dead they give life; when bound, they enable one to rise in the air.

मनःस्थैर्यं स्थिरो वायुस्ततो बिन्दुः स्थिरो भवेत् ।
बिन्दुस्थैर्यात् सदा सत्त्वं पिण्डस्थैर्यं प्रजायते ॥ २८ ॥

(28) *When the mind is steady, the prāṇa is also steady, and hence is the stability of seminal fluid; by the steadiness of the seminal fluid, there arises purity and stability of the body.*

इन्द्रियाणां मनो नाथो मनोनाथस्तु मारुतः ।
मारुतस्य लयो नाथः स लयो नादमाश्रितः ॥ २९ ॥

(29) *The mind is superior to sense organs. Prāṇa is the lord of the mind. Laya (or absorption) of prāṇa is superior, and that laya depends on the nāda (the inner sounds).*

सोऽयमेवास्तु मोक्षाख्यो मास्तु वापि मतान्तरे ।
मनः प्राणलये कश्चिदानन्दः सम्प्रवर्तते ॥ ३० ॥

(30) *This itself is considered mokṣa (liberation), though others say that it is not. However, when the prāṇa and the mind have been absorbed, an indefinable ānanda ensues.*

प्रनष्टश्वासनिश्वासः प्रध्वस्तविषयग्रहः ।
निश्चेष्टो निर्विकारश्च लयो जयति योगिनाम् ॥ ३१ ॥

(31) *When there is suspension of inhaling and exhaling, then the attractions towards sense objects are destroyed; when there is no activity of the mind*

and body, the yogī obtains success in absorption (laya).

उच्छिन्नसर्वसङ्कल्पो निःशेषाशेषचेष्टितः ।
स्वावगम्यो लयः कोऽपि जायते वाग्गोचरः ॥ ३२ ॥

(32) When both mental and physical activities cease, the indescribable state of laya ensues, which can only be realized intuitively and cannot be described by words.

यत्र दृष्टिर्लयस्तत्र भूतेन्द्रियसनातनी ।
सा शक्तिर्जीवभूतानां द्वे अलक्ष्ये लयं गते ॥ ३३ ॥

(33) Where there is vision (mental perception), there is laya (absorption in Brahman). Then that (avidyā) in beings which exists eternally in the senses and the elements, and the energy (Śakti) which is in all living beings, are absorbed in the indefinable.

लयो लय इति प्राहुः कीदृधं: लयलक्षणम् ।
अपुनर्वासनोत्थानाल्लयो विषयविस्मृतिः ॥ ३४ ॥

(34) People keep repeating laya, laya; but how is it defined? Laya is the non-recollection of the objects of the senses due to the non-recurrence of vāsanas.

वेदशास्त्रपुराणानि सामान्यगणिका इव ।
एकैव शाम्भवी मुद्रा गुप्ता कुलवधूरिव ॥ ३५ ॥

(35) *The Vedas, Śāstras and Purāṇas are like the courtesans (as they are available to all men). But Śāmbhavī mudrā is to be guarded like a respectable well-born woman.*

अन्तर्लक्ष्यं   बहिर्दृष्टिर्निमेषोन्मेषवर्जिता ।
एषा सा शाम्भवी मुद्रा वेदशास्त्रेषु गोपिता ॥ ३६ ॥

(36) *When there is concentration on an internal object, and the outward sight is devoid of winking, it is called Śāmbhavīmudrā. It is hidden in the Vedas and Śāstras.*

अन्तर्लक्ष्यविलीनचित्तपवनो योगी यदा वर्तते ।
        दृष्ट्या निश्चलतारया बहिरधः पश्यन्नपश्यन्नपि ।
मुद्रेयं खलु शाम्भवी भवति सा लब्धा प्रसादाद् गुरोः ।
        शून्याशून्यविलक्षणं स्फुरित तत्त्वं पदं शाम्भवम् ॥ ३७ ॥

(37) *When the yogī remains with the mind and breath absorbed in the internal object, when the pupils of the eye are without movement, and even when they are apparently looking outside, the eyes do not actually grasp the objects; that is indeed called the Śāmbhavī mudrā. That is obtained by the grace of the guru. Then the yogī realizes the state of Śambhu, which is resplendent and which is beyond Śūnyāśūnya (void and non-void).*

श्री शाम्भव्याश्च खेचर्या अवस्थाधामभेदतः ।
भवेच्चित्तलयानन्दः शून्ये चित्सुखरूपिणि ॥ ३८ ॥

(38) The Śāmbhavī and Khecarī mudrās, though differing in the position of the eyes and places, are one in their result. Both of them bring about the state of ānanda, absorption of the mind in the void which is of the nature of Citsukha (Brahman).

तारे ज्योतिषिसंयोज्य किञ्चिदुन्नमयेद्भ्रुवौ ।
पूर्वयोगं मनो युञ्जन्नुन्मनीकारकः क्षणात् ॥ ३९ ॥

(39) Direct the pupils (of the eyes) towards the light by raising the eyebrows a little upwards. Concentrating the mind on the earlier mentioned yoga practice, the Unmanī-avasthā comes about immediately.

केचिदागमजालेन   केचिन्निगमसङ्कुलैः ।
केचित्तर्केण मुह्यन्ति नैव जानन्ति तारकम् ॥ ४० ॥

(40) Some confuse themselves by Āgamas and some by Nigamas and others by logic. They do not know that which gives them freedom.

अर्धोन्मीलितलोचनः स्थिरमना नासाग्रदत्तेक्षण-
    श्चन्द्राकार्विप   लीनतामुपनयन्निष्पन्दभावेन यः ।
ज्योतीरूपमशेषबीजमखिलं देदीप्यमानं परं
    तत्त्वं तत्पदमेति वस्तु परमं वाच्यं किमत्राधिकम् ॥ ४१ ॥

(41) With half-closed eyes fixed on the tip of the nose, with a steadied mind, and with the sun and the moon reduced to the state of suspension (by directing the

prāṇa from iḍā and piṅgalā, and forcing it into suṣumnā), the yogī attains that state wherein he experiences the Supreme Reality in the form of resplendent light (jyoti), which is the source of all things, and which is the most supreme object to be gained. What else higher than this could be expected?

दिवा न पूजयेल्लिङ्गं रात्रौ चैव न पूजयेत्।
सर्वदा पूजयेल्लिङ्गं दिवारात्रिनिरोधतः ॥ ४२ ॥

(42) Do not worship the liṅga (ātman) in the day and in the night (alone). Stopping the day and the night, the liṅga should be worshipped constantly.

सव्यदक्षिणनडीस्थो मध्ये चरति मारुतः।
तिष्ठते खेचरी मुद्रा तस्मिन्स्थाने न संशयः ॥ ४३ ॥

(43) Khecarīmudrā: When the prāṇa which naturally flows through the right and the left nāḍīs moves in the middle, khecarī becomes steady. There is no doubt about this.

इडापिङ्गलयोर्मध्ये शून्यं चैवानिलं ग्रसेत्।
तिष्ठते खेचरी मुद्रा तत्र सत्यं पुनः पुनः ॥ ४४ ॥

(44) When the void between iḍā and piṅgalā swallows the breath, then the khecarī mudrā becomes steady. This is the correct method without doubt.

सूर्याचन्द्रमसोर्मध्ये निरालम्बान्तरे पुनः।
संस्थिता व्योमचक्रे या सा मुद्रा नाम खेचरी ॥ ४५ ॥

(45) In the middle of the unsupported space between the iḍā and piṅgalā, the vyomacakra is situated. The mudrā practiced in this space is called the khecarī mudrā.

सोमाद्यत्रोदिता धारा साक्षात्सा शिववल्लभा।
पूरयेदतुलां दिव्यां सुषुम्नां पश्चिमे मुखे॥ ४६ ॥

(46) The khecarī mudrā in which the stream of nectar flows from the moon, is very much liked by Lord Śiva. The suṣumnā, having no equal, is the best of the nāḍīs which must be closed at the rear end of the mouth (by the tongue).

पुरस्ताच्चैव पूर्येत निश्चिता खेचरी भवेत्।
अभ्यस्ता खेचरी मुद्राप्युन्मनी संप्रजायते॥ ४७ ॥

(47) If the prāṇa is stopped in the front as well, then khecarī definitely comes into being. By frequent practice of khecarī, the Unmanī comes into being.

भ्रवोर्मध्ये शिवस्थानं मनस्तत्र विलीयते।
ज्ञातव्यं तत्पदं तुर्यं तत्र कालो न विद्यते॥ ४८ ॥

(48) Between the eyebrows, which is the seat of Lord Śiva, the mind becomes absorbed. This is known as the fourth state (turīya) where there is suspension of time.

अभ्यसेत् खेचरीं तावद्यावत्स्याद्योगनिद्रित:।
सम्प्राप्तयोगनिद्रस्य कालो नास्ति कदाचन॥ ४९ ॥

(49) One should practice Khecarī mudrā until he gets into the Yoganidrā. When Yoganidrā is obtained there is no death.

निरालम्बं मनः कृत्वा न किञ्चिदपि चिन्तयेत् ।
स बाह्याभ्यन्तरे व्योम्नि घटवत्तिष्ठति ध्रुवम् ॥५०॥

(50) After making the mind supportless (by removing it from every object of conception), he should not think of anything. He certainly then remains like a pot filled inside and outside with ākāśa.

बाह्यवायुर्यथा लीनस्तथा मध्यो न संशयः ।
स्वस्थाने स्थिरतामेति पवनो मनसा सह ॥५१॥

(51) When the outside breath from without ceases, the breath within the body also becomes absorbed. There is no doubt about it. After this the prāṇa, along with the mind, becomes steady in its own position.

एवमभ्यस्यतस्तस्य वायुमार्गे दिवानिशम् ।
अभ्यासाज्जीर्यते वायुर्मनस्तत्रैव लीयते ॥५२॥

(52) By thus practicing restraint of prāṇa night and day, the prāṇa through practice is absorbed; then the mind is also abosrbed.

अमृतैः प्लावयेद्देहमापादतलमस्तकम् ।
सिद्ध्यत्येव महाकायो महाबलपराक्रमः ॥५३॥

(53) One should saturate the body from head to foot with the stream of nectar (flowing from the Moon).

He then becomes endowed with an excellent body, great strength, and valor. Thus khecarī has been described.

शक्तिमध्ये मनः कृत्वा शक्तिं मानसमध्यगाम् ।
मनसा मन आलोक्य धारयेत्परमं पदम् ॥५४॥

(54) *Placing the mind in the Śakti (Kuṇḍalinī), and placing the Śakti in the center of the mind, and observing the mind with the mind, meditate on the Supreme state.*

खमध्ये कुरु चात्मानमात्ममध्ये च खं कुरु ।
सर्वं च खमयं कृत्वा न किञ्चिदपि चिन्तयेत् ॥५५॥

(55) *Place Ātman in the midst of ākāśa, and the ākāśa in the midst of Ātman. And converting everything into ākāśa, one must not think of anything else.*

अन्तः शून्यो बहिः शून्यः शून्यः कुम्भ इवाम्बरे ।
अन्तः पूर्णो बहिः पूर्णः पूर्णः कुम्भ इवार्णवे ॥५६॥

(56) *Void within and void without, he is like an empty pot in ākāśa (full within and full without). He is like a full pot in the ocean, full within and full without.*

बाह्यचिन्ता न कर्त्तव्या तथैवान्तरचिन्तनम् ।
सर्वचिन्तां परित्यज्य न किञ्चिदपि चिन्तयेत् ॥५७॥

(57) He should cease thinking of anything external.
Neither should he be thinking of anything within.
Abandoning all thoughts he should dwell on nothing.

संकल्पमात्रकलनैव जगत्समग्रं
संकल्पमात्रकलनैव मनोविलास: ।
संकल्पमात्रमतिमुत्सृज निर्विकल्प–
माश्रित्य निश्चयमवाप्नुहि राम शान्तिम् ॥ ५८ ॥

(58) The external universe is created merely by our
thoughts, as also the imaginary world. Giving up all
thoughts that are imaginary and resorting to
nirvikalpa (samādhi) O Rāma, you will find peace.
(From Yogavāsiṣṭha).

कर्पूरमनले यद्वत्सैन्धवं सलिले यथा।
तथा सन्धीयमानं च मनस्तत्त्वे विलीयते ॥ ५९ ॥

(59) As camphor disappears when burnt, and as salt
dissolves in water, the concentrating mind merges with
the object of meditation.

ज्ञेयं सर्वं प्रतीतं च ज्ञानं च मन उच्यते।
ज्ञानं ज्ञेयं समं नष्टं नान्य: पन्था द्वितीयक: ॥ ६० ॥

(60) Everything that is seen can be known and what
is known, as well as knowledge, is called the mind.
When the known and the knowledge are lost, there is
no second path (to mokṣa).

मनोदृश्यमिदं सर्वं यत्किञ्चित्सचराचरम् ।
मनसो ह्युन्मनीभावाद् द्वैतं नैवोपलभ्यते ॥ ६१ ॥

(61) Both animate and inanimate things in the universe are perceived by the mind. When the mind is lost in the Unmanī state, then duality is not experienced.

ज्ञेयवस्तुपरित्यागाद् विलयं याति मानसम् ।
मनसो विलये जाते कैवल्यमवशिष्यते ॥ ६२ ॥

(62) By the abandonment of all objects, the mind reaches the state of absorption. When the mind gets absorbed, kaivalya alone remains.

एवं नानाविधोपायाः सम्यक्स्वानुभवान्विताः ।
समाधिमार्गाः कथिताः पूर्वाचार्यैर्महात्मभिः ॥ ६३ ॥

(63) These are the various paths and means for attaining samādhi, described by the great ancient teachers from their own experience.

सुषुम्नायै कुण्डलिन्यै सुधायै चन्द्रजन्मने ।
मनोन्मन्यै नमस्तुभ्यं महाशक्त्यै चिदात्मने ॥ ६४ ॥

(64) Salutations to the suṣumnā, to the kuṇḍalinī, to Sudhā that arises in the moon, to the manonmanī, and to the Great Power of the Ātman in the form of pure consciousness.

अशक्यतत्त्वबोधानां मूढानामपि सम्मतम् ।
प्रोक्तं गोरक्षनाथेन नादोपासनमुज्यते ॥ ६५ ॥

(65) I shall describe nādopāsana taught by Gorakṣanātha. This is suitable even for those of inferior intellect who are not capable of realising the supreme truth.

श्री आदिनाथेन सपादकोटिलयप्रकारा: कथिता जयन्ति ।
नादानुसन्धानकमेकमेव मन्यामहे मुख्यतमं लयानाम् ॥ ६६ ॥

(66) Śrī Ādinātha (Lord Śiva) has given one crore and a quarter (1,25,00,000) of ways for the attainment of laya, but we consider nādopāsana the best of all layas.

मुक्तासने स्थितो योगी मुद्रां सन्धाय शाम्भवीम् ।
शृणुयाद् दक्षिणे कर्णे नादमन्त:स्थमेकधी: ॥ ६७ ॥

(67) The yogī sitting in the muktāsana and assuming the śāmbhavī mudrā, should listen with a concentrated mind to the sounds within. These are heard in the right ear.

श्रवणपुटनयनयुगलघ्राणमुखानां निरोधनं कार्यम् ।
शुद्धसुषुम्नासरणौ स्फुटममल: श्रूयते नाद: ॥ ६८ ॥

(68) Close the ears, the nose, the mouth and the eyes. Then a clear sound is heard distinctly in the suṣumnā which has been purified.

आरम्भश्च घटश्चैव तथा परिचयोऽपि च।
निष्पत्ति: सर्वयोगेषु स्यादवस्थाचतुष्टयम्॥ ६९ ॥

*(69) In all the yogic practices there are four stages:
ārambha, ghaṭa, paricaya, and niṣpatti.*

ब्रह्मग्रन्थेर्भवेद्   भेदो ह्यानन्द: शून्यसम्भव:।
विचित्र: क्वणको देहेऽनाहत: श्रूयते ध्वनि:॥ ७० ॥

*(70) Ārambhāvasthā: (In the first stage), there
is the breaking open of Brahmagranthi (knot
of Brahma that is in the Anāhata-cakra). Then,
there is bliss which arises from the void.
Simultaneously, the various sweet tinkling sounds
(as of ornaments) and the unstruck sound anāhata-
dhvani (arising from the ākāśa in the heart), are
heard in the body.*

दिव्यदेहश्च तेजस्वी दिव्यगन्धस्त्वरोगवान्।
सम्पूर्णहृदय: शून्य आरम्भे योगवान् भवेत्॥ ७१ ॥

*(71) In the ārambhāvasthā, the yogī has his heart
full (of bliss) and he gets a lustrous body; he is
radiant and emits a sweet smell and is free of all
diseases.*

द्वितीयायां घटीकृत्य वायुर्भवति मध्यग:।
दृढासनो भवेद् योगी ज्ञानी देवसमस्तदा॥ ७२ ॥

*(72) Ghaṭāvasthā: In the second stage, the prāṇa
unites (with apāna, nāda and bindu) and enters the*

middle region. The yogī then becomes firm in the āsanas, his intellect becomes more keen, and he becomes equal to the devas.

विष्णुग्रन्थेस्ततो   भेदात् परमानन्दसूचकः ।
अतिशून्ये विमर्दश्च भेरीशब्दस्तथा भवेत् ॥ ७३ ॥

(73) When Viṣṇugranthi in the supreme void is pierced, it is indicative of great bliss. Then there is a rumbling sound like that of a kettledrum.

तृतीयायां तु विज्ञेयो विहायोमर्दलध्वनिः ।
महाशून्यं   तदायाति सर्वसिद्धिसमाश्रयम् ॥ ७४ ॥

(74) Paricayāvasthā: In the third stage, a sound like that of mardala is heard in the ākāśa (lying between the eyebrows). The vāyu (the prāṇa) goes to the mahāśūnya, which is the seat of all siddhis.

चित्तानन्दं तदा जित्वा सहजानन्दसम्भवः ।
दोषदुःखजराव्याधिक्षुधानिद्राविवर्जितः ॥ ७५ ॥

(75) Having overcome the blissful state of the mind, the yogī experiences the natural state of bliss. He then becomes free from all faults, pains, old age, diseases, hunger, and sleep.

रुद्रग्रन्थिं यदा भित्त्वा शर्वपीठगतोऽनिलः ।
निष्पत्तौ वैणवः शब्दः क्वणद्वीणाक्वणे भवेत् ॥ ७६ ॥

(76) Niṣpatti-avasthā: In niṣpatti-avasthā, when the prāṇa pierces the rudragranthi (existing at the ājñā cakra), it goes to the seat of Īśvara. Then is heard the sound of the flute which assumes the resonance of the veena.

एकीभूतं तदा चित्तं राजयोगाभिधानकम् ।
सृष्टिसंहारकर्त्तासौ   योगीश्वरसमो भवेत् ॥ ७७ ॥

(77) When the mind becomes one (with the object concentrated upon), it is called Rājayoga. At that stage the yogī being the master of creation and destruction, becomes the equal of Īśvara.

अस्तु वा मास्तु वा मुक्तिरत्रैवाखण्डितं सुखम् ।
लयोद्भवमिदं   सौख्यं   राजयोगादवाप्यते ॥ ७८ ॥

(78) Let there be mukti or not, here is uninterrupted Bliss. The bliss arising from laya is obtained only from the practice of Rājayoga.

राजयोगमजानन्तः   केवलं हठकर्मिणः ।
एतानभ्यासिनो मन्ये प्रयासफलवर्जितान् ॥ ७९ ॥

(79) Those who do not understand Rājayoga and only practice Haṭhakarma, such practioners, I think, are cheated of the fruits of their efforts.

उन्मन्यवाप्तये   शीघ्रं भ्रू ध्यानं मम सम्मतम् ।
राजयोगपदं प्राप्तुं सुखोपायोऽल्पचेतसाम् ।
सद्यः प्रत्ययसन्धायी जायते नादजो लयः ॥ ८० ॥

(80) *I think that contemplation on the space between the eyebrows is the best way for the attainment of the Unmanī-avasthā in a short time. For people of inferior intellect, the absorption brought about by nāda (yoga) which gives immediate experience is an easy means to attain the state of Rājayoga.*

नादानुसन्धानसमाधिभाजां योगीश्वराणां हृदि वर्धमानम् ।
आनन्दमेकं वचसामगम्यं जानाति तं श्रीगुरुनाथ एक: ॥ ८१ ॥

(81) *Great yogis, who practice samādhi through the concentration on nāda, experience a joy arising in their hearts that surpasses all description, which only Śrī Gurunātha (supreme teacher) is able to know.*

कर्णौ पिधाय हस्ताभ्यां यं शृणोति ध्वनिं मुनि: ।
तत्र चित्तं स्थिरीकुर्याद्यावत्स्थिरपदं व्रजेत् ॥ ८२ ॥

(82) *The muni who hears the sounds when he closes his ears with his two hands should fix his mind on it until he attains the steady state.*

अभ्यस्यमानो नादोऽयं बाह्यमावृणुते ध्वनिम् ।
पक्षाद्विक्षेपमखिलं जित्वा योगी सुखी भवेत् ॥ ८३ ॥

(83) *This (anāhata) sound which one listens to, gradually overpowers and drowns out the external sounds. The yogī, overcoming the instability of his mind will, in fifteen days, become contented and happy.*

श्रूयते प्रथमाभ्यासे नादो नानाविधो महान् ।
ततोऽभ्यासे वर्धमाने श्रूयते सूक्ष्मसूक्ष्मकः ॥८४॥

(84) During the initial stages of the practice, various prominent, inner sounds are heard. But when progress is made, they become more and more subtle.

आदौ   जलधिजीमूतभेरीझर्झरसम्भवाः ।
मध्ये मर्दलशङ्खोत्था घण्टाकाहलजास्तथा ॥८५॥

(85) In the beginning, the sounds resemble those of the ocean, the clouds, the kettledrum, and jarjara (a sort of drum cymbal). In the middle they resemble those arising from the mardala, the conch, the bell, and the horn.

अन्ते तु किङ्किणीवंशवीणाभ्रमरनिःस्वनाः ।
इति   नानाविधा नादाः श्रूयन्ते देहमध्यगाः ॥८६॥

(86) In the end they resemble those of the tinkling bells, the flute, the veena, and the bees. Thus are heard the various sounds from the middle of the body.

महति श्रूयमाणेऽपि मेघभेर्यादिके ध्वनौ ।
तत्र   सूक्ष्मात्सूक्ष्मतरं नादमेव परामृशेत् ॥८७॥

(87) Even when the loud sounds resembling those of the clouds and the kettle drum are heard, he should try to fix his attention on the subtler than the subtle sounds alone.

घनमुत्सृज्य वा सूक्ष्मे सूक्ष्ममुत्सृज्य वा घने।
रममाणमपि क्षिप्तं मनो नान्यत्र चालयेत्॥ ८८॥

*(88) Even though his attention changes from the loud
to the subtle sounds or from subtle to loud, he should
never allow his attention to wander to other
extraneous sounds.*

यत्र कुत्रापि वा नादे लगति प्रथमं मनः।
तत्रैव सुस्थिरीभूय तेन सार्धं विलीयते॥ ८९॥

*(89) In whatever inner sound the mind first focuses
itself, in that it reaches steadiness, and becomes one
with it in the end.*

मकरन्दं पिबन् भृङ्गो गन्धं नापेक्षते यथा।
नादासक्तं तथा चित्तं विषयान्न हि काङ्क्षते॥ १०॥

*(90) As a bee, through drinking nectar of flowers,
cares not for the fragrance, so the mind absorbed in
the nāda does not care for the objects of enjoyment.*

मनो मत्तगजेन्द्रस्य विषयोद्यानचारिणः।
नियन्त्रणे समर्थोऽयं निनादनिशिताङ्कुशः॥ ९१॥

*(91) The sharp iron goad of nāda can effectively curb
the mind which behaves like a mad elephant that
wanders in the garden of the sense objects.*

बद्धं तु नादबन्धेन मनः संत्यक्तचापलम्।
प्रयाति सुतरां स्थैर्यं छिन्नपक्षः खगो यथा॥ ९२॥

(92) When the mind is bound by the sounds of nāda, and has given up its fickleness, then it attains excellent steadiness (and) it is like a bird that has lost its wings.

सर्वचिन्तां परित्यज्य सावधानेन चेतसा।
नाद एवानुसन्धेयो योगसाम्राज्यमिच्छता॥ ९३॥

(93) The yogī, desirous of obtaining the sovereignty of yoga, should abandon all thoughts, and with a carefully concentrated mind, should meditate on the nāda alone.

नादोऽन्तरङ्गसारङ्गबन्धेन वागुरायते।
अन्तरङ्गकुरङ्गस्य वधे व्याधायतेऽपि च॥ ९४॥

(94) Nāda is like a snare for catching the deer within, i.e., the mind. It is also the hunter who kills the deer (the mind).

अन्तरङ्गस्य यमिनो वाजिनः परिघायते।
नादोपास्तिरतो नित्यमवधार्या हि योगिना॥ ९५॥

(95) (Nāda) is like the bolt of a stable that prevents horses in the form of the mind of the yogī from wandering. A yogī therefore should daily practice concentration upon the nāda.

बद्धं विमुक्तचाञ्चल्यं नादगन्धकजारणात्।
मनः पारदमाप्नोति निरालम्बाख्यखेऽटनम्॥ ९६॥

(96) Mercury, calcinated by the action of sulfur, becomes solidified and gives up its restlessness and rises in the air. Similarly, the mind concentrating on the nāda, gives up its fickleness and roams in the supportless ākāśa.

नादश्रवणतः   क्षिप्रमन्तरङ्गभुजङ्गमः ।
विस्मृत्य सर्वमेकाग्रः कुत्रचिन्न हि धावति ॥ ९७ ॥

(97) The mind, like a serpent within, hearing the sound of nāda, forgets everything and becomes one pointed and does not run away.

काष्ठे प्रतर्त्तितो वह्निः काष्ठेन सह शाम्यति ।
नादे   प्रवर्त्तितं चित्तं नादेन सह लीयते ॥ ९८ ॥

(98) The fire that burns a piece of wood, dies along with the wood. So also the mind engaged in nāda gets absorbed along with nāda.

घण्टादिनादसक्तस्तब्धान्तःकरणहरिणस्य ।
प्रहरणमपि सुकरं शरसन्धानप्रवीणश्चेत् ॥ ९९ ॥

(99) A skillful archer can easily kill a deer when it stands, attracted by the sounds of bells etc., so also, the deer in the form of the mind (for a skillful yogī).

अनाहतस्य   शब्दस्य ध्वनिर्य उपलभ्यते ।
ध्वनेरन्तर्गतं ज्ञेयं ज्ञेयस्यान्तर्गतं   मनः ।
मनस्तत्र लयं याति तद्विष्णोः परमं पदम् ॥ १०० ॥

(100) *That which is to be known lies inside the dhvani which is the anāhata sound; and the mind is within that which is to be known (Supreme Self). The mind gets absorbed therein; that is the supreme state of Viṣṇu.*

तावदाकाशसङ्कल्पो यावच्छब्द: प्रवर्तते ।
नि:शब्दं तत्परं ब्रह्म परमात्मेति गीयते ॥ १०१ ॥

(101) *The conception of ākāśa (the generation of sound) exists as long as the sound is heard. The soundless state is praised as Parabrahman or Paramātman.*

यत् किञ्चिन्नादरूपेण श्रूयते शक्तिरेव सा ।
यस्तत्त्वान्तो निराकार: स एव परमेश्वर: ॥१०२॥

(102) *Whatever is heard in the form of nāda is only Śakti. The supreme truth is without form. That itself is Parameśvara.*

सर्वे हठलयोपाया राजयोगस्य सिद्धये ।
राजयोगसमारूढ: पुरुष: कालवञ्चक: ॥१०३॥

(103) *All the Haṭha and Laya Yoga practices are only for the attainment of Rājayoga. Those perfected in Rājayoga cheat death.*

तत्त्वं बीजं हठ: क्षेत्रमौदासीन्यं जलं त्रिभि: ।
उन्मनी कल्पलतिका सद्य एव प्रवर्तते ॥ १०४ ॥

(104) Mind is the seed, Haṭhayoga is the soil, and extreme vairāgya is the water. By these three, the kalpa creeper (that gives whatever is desired), the Unmanī (Turīya avasthā) springs up quickly.

सदा नादानुसन्धानात् क्षीयन्ते पापसञ्चया: ।
निरञ्जने विलीयेते निश्चितं चित्तमारुतौ ॥ १०५ ॥

(105) By constant practice of concentration on Nāda, all vices are destroyed. The mind and the prāṇa verily get absorbed in that pure state (caitanya).

शंखदुन्दुभिनादं च न शृणोति कदाचन।
काष्ठवज्जायते देह उन्मन्यावस्थया ध्रुवम् ॥ १०६ ॥

(106) During Unmanī-avasthā the body becomes like a log of wood. The yogī hears nothing, not even the (loud) sounds of a conch or dundubhi (a large drum).

सर्वावस्थाविनिर्मुक्त: सर्वचिन्ताविवर्जित: ।
मृतवत्तिष्ठते योगी स मुक्तो नात्र संशय: ॥ १०७ ॥

(107) The yogī, who has passed beyond all states and is not troubled by any thoughts (or memories), remains like one dead. Undoubtedly he is a mukta, emancipated while living (jīvanmukta).

खाद्यते न च कालेन बाध्यते न च कर्मणा।
साध्यते न स केनापि योगी युक्त: समाधिना ॥ १०८ ॥

(108) The yogī in samādhi is not swallowed up by the

process of Time (death). He is not influenced by good or bad karma, nor is he affected by anything done against him.

न गन्धं न रसं रूपं न च स्पर्शं न निःस्वनम् ।
नात्मानं न परं वेत्ति योगी युक्तः समाधिना ॥ १०९ ॥

(109) The yogī in samādhi experiences neither smell, taste, touch, sound, shape nor color. He is not aware of himself or the others.

चित्तं न सुसं नो जाग्रत्स्मृतिविस्मृतिवर्जितम् ।
न चास्तमेति नोदेति यस्यासौ मुक्त एव सः ॥ ११० ॥

(110) He is certainly a jīvanmukta (liberated while still living) when his consciousness is neither asleep nor awake, when his citta is free from smṛti (memory) or vismṛti (forgetfulness), and when he is neither dead nor living.

न विजानाति शीतोष्णं न दुःखं न सुखं तथा ।
न मानं नापमानं च योगी युक्तः समाधिना ॥ १११ ॥

(111) The yogī in samādhi is not affected by heat or cold, pain or pleasure, honor or disgrace.

स्वस्थो जाग्रदवस्थायां सुप्तवद्योऽवतिष्ठते ।
निःश्वासोच्छ्वासहीनश्च निश्चतं मुक्त एव सः ॥ ११२ ॥

(112) In the waking state, when a yogī stays, as if asleep, in a steady state devoid of inhalation and

exhalation, then indeed is he liberated.

अवध्यः सर्वशस्त्राणामशक्यः सर्वदेहिनाम् ।
अग्राह्यो मन्त्रयन्त्राणां योगी युक्तः समाधिना ॥ ११३ ॥

(113) The yogī in samādhi cannot be killed by any weapon; all the world cannot overpower him. He is beyond the powers of mantras and yantras.

यावन्नैव प्रविशति चरन्मारुतो मध्यमार्गे,
यावद्बिन्दुर्न भवति दृढ:प्राणवातप्रबन्धात् ।
यावद्ध्याने सहजसदृशं जायते नैव तत्त्वं,
ताज्ज्ञानं वदति तदिदं दम्भमिथ्याप्रलाप: ॥ ११४ ॥

इति हठयोगप्रदीपिकायां समाधिलक्षणं नाम चतुर्थोपदेश: ॥

(114) As long as the prāṇa does not enter the middle path (suṣumnā), as long as the bindu (semen) does not become solid from the restraint of breath, as long as the mind (citta) does not become of the same nature as the object contemplated upon (Brahman) during meditation - so long are those who merely talk of jñana nothing but vain talkers and untruthful men.

Thus ends the fourth chapter of *Haṭha Yoga Pradīpīkā* called Samādhilakṣaṇa

Krishna says in the **Bhagavatam**, "There are only three ways to liberation laid down by me. They are: jnana, karma, and bhakti." Then why is [Raja] Yoga said to be the chief means of attaining liberation? The answer is that all three are combined in the eight-fold Yoga.

The sruti says, "The Self alone is to be seen, heard, contemplated upon and realized." That Self can be attained by sravana (listening), manana (reflection), and nididhyasana (realization). The first two are included in swadhyaya, which is one of the subdivisions of niyama, the second stage of Yoga. Swadhyaya is the thorough study of the teachings on liberation, with a complete knowledge of their inner meanings and symbolism. Nididhyasana is the restraining of the ideal that there is anything else besides Brahman, and the fostering of the realization that everything is Brahman. This is contained in dhyana, the seventh stage of [Raja] Yoga.

Karma Yoga, which is performing all acts as an offering to Ishwara, is contained in the Kriya Yoga described by Patanjali. Patanjali says, "Kriya Yoga is tapas, swadhyaya, and Ishwara pranidhana." Tapas means the purification of the body by the observance of various penances. Swadhyaya consists of those studies that bring about a predominance of the sattva guna. Ishwara pranidhana is praising Ishwara, remembering and worshipping him by word, thought and action, and an unswerving devotion to him.

Bhakti really means the constant perception of the form of the Lord by the inner organ. There are nine kinds of bhakti: hearing the lore concerning the Lord, singing it, remembering Him, worshipping His feet, offering flowers to Him, bowing to Him (in spirit), regarding oneself as His servant, becoming His companion and wholly offering oneself to Him. These are all included in Ishwara pranidhana. Bhakti has been described by Narayana Tirtha as an unbroken stream of love towards the feet of the Lord - a love that is the be all and end all of a person's existence, and during which he is, as it were, absorbed in the object of his devotion. Madhusudana Saraswati has also described it as a state of mind, when previous to its being utterly annihilated and absorbed, it becomes of a nature of the Lord. Thus Bhakti, in its most transcendental aspect, is included in Samprajnata samadhi.

So the three ways laid down by Krishna in the **Bhagavatam** have been shown to be included in the stages of Yoga. Thus Yoga practiced in its entiretly, and in the order laid down, is enough for the attainment of liberation. In this sense alone are to be understood the words in the Puranas saying that Brahman is to be attained by Yoga.

Epilogue

Address delivered by Swami Vishnudevananda at the Final Ceremony of the Yoga Sadhana Intensive at the Sivananda Ashram Yoga Camp during June, 1987

As many of you know, the *Hatha Yoga Pradipika* is the original treatise on Hatha Yoga. It was written down by Swami Svatmarama, whose name means "he who is sporting with his own Atman." We, on the other hand, are "Bhogaramas," because we sport with our own senses.

Modern Hatha Yoga has been developed and enlarged from Svatmarama's book. There are three other classical treatises on Hatha Yoga: the *Siva Samhita, Gherandha Samhita,* and the *Goraksha Samhita.* They are all within the tradition of Ashtanga Yoga (the eight-limbed Yoga). Raja Yoga, Hatha Yoga, Kundalini Yoga, Laya Yoga, Mantra Yoga are all part of Ashtanga Yoga. They differ a little bit only in approach.

Of the eight steps of Ashtanga Yoga, yama and niyama are common to all these Yogas. Asanas (or postures) were not elaborated on too much by some of these treatises; Patanjali's *Yoga Sutras* is an example. He describes only one asana, saying only that sitting comfortably in a pose is asana. He did not elaborate beyond that because in those days people were practicing cultural poses in their daily lives as part of the Gurukhula system of education.

Under the Gurukhula system, a student goes to live under the guidance of a teacher for ten to twelve years. The teacher might have thirty or forty students. He would have a little plot of land and simple accommodations, a few cows or other cattle for their livelihood. The students would help in tilling the land, cultivating, and milking the cows. In return, the teacher would impart his knowledge. Part of the knowledge imparted was that of asanas and pranayama; they were given to all, beginners as well as advanced students. Every child had to perform pranayama with the Gayatri mantra.

Yama and niyama (ethics and morals), were all practiced in daily life. Hatha yogis elaborated on the regulations concerning cleanliness, not only by cleaning the teeth and the rest of the body, but going even deeper - cleaning the nasal passages, the stomach, etc. And even further, into advanced cleaning through pranayama and through the Bija mantras of the elements. For example, the Bija mantra of earth is Lam, Vam is the Bija mantra for water, Ram is the Bija mantra for fire, Tam is the Bija mantra for the moon. Gross matter of any kind is called earth, any liquid is water, any fire is called Ram, and any energy which cools the body and brings purification is called Tam, or moon, or nectar. So, by using various Bija mantras, you are purifying the system through subtle pranayama. In the Gurukhula system there was the practice of such things as Bija mantras, so there was no need for Patanjali or other Raja yogis to describe them. Students learned these practices directly from the teacher.

Although asanas were not elaborated on by Patanjali and other Raja yogis, they were performed to cause the body to become very still. The cultural poses trained the body so that it could be kept still and steady without strain or effort. When such a pose is found - one that is easy and comfortable for you - stick to it all of your life. You will get rock-like firmness, and your nerve energy will start flowing when you use it for meditation. Your metabolic activity, breathing mechanism, pulse rate, and blood pressure will go down. As these metabolic activities slow down when you sit quietly, you attain the first step of Raja Yoga.

Then you go to the second level, pranayama. Again, Patanjali only says this much: that regulation of inhalation and exhalation is pranayama. Its purpose is to reduce the velocity of the mind. People were practicing other pranayamas: Anuloma Viloma, Bhastrika, Ujjayi, Surya bedha - so they understood that prana is not the physical air. They learned these techniques also from the guru, as it was part of their daily routine. That is why Raja Yoga had no need to go into detail; Patanjali didn't have to elaborate on it as it was common knowledge. Only later on, when people's minds began wandering because they no longer had the discipline, and the Gurukhula system declined, then at that time Swatmarama introduced Hatha Yoga. It is for the same end as Raja Yoga, but it now has to explain those asanas and pranayamas which had been taught as part of the Gurukhula system.

The fourth step is pratyahara or withdrawal of the mind from the senses, or introversion. Patanjali says, "*Yoga chitta vritti nirodha.*" Yoga is stilling the mental modifications of the mind. Raja Yoga elaborated these three processes, and so did Svatmarama Yogi, but in a way that gave more control. Most people, by merely closing their eyes, cannot regulate their thoughts. But when they perform pranayama, mudras or bandhas properly, then the prana moves in the Sushumna, causing the mind to become very still. Raja Yoga does not say how to achieve this mental state except through stopping the mind. The teacher would also have taught the student how to perform bandhas and mudras in the Gurukhula system, so Patanjali only gives the theory of concentration and samyama.

Samyama is concentration, meditation, and samadhi; they are only varying amounts of mental control. Concentration's quality is less, in meditation quality is a little better. In meditation, your mind is pure like a candle which is steady when there is no wind. Patanjali says that you can do samyama on anything, using these three processes, and get the knowledge of that particular element. Suppose you are concentrating on Lam (in the Muladhara chakra, representing the earth element), then earth won't affect you; you will have power over earth, solid matter. Raja Yoga explains the theory, but Hatha Yoga puts it into practice. And that is the intense sadhana described in these pages.

They are almost the same activities I performed when I was in the Himalayas undergoing my own training. With Gurudev's Grace and with His blessings, I went to Uttarkashi and I followed this same program. Morning, midday, evening, and midnight I practiced pranayama, asanas, bandhas, plus about 200 malas of mantra (taking about three or four hours). I had hardly two or three hours of sleep each night, but that was sufficient for the body. It doesn't need too much because intense energy starts flowing. You can experience these things.

With God's Grace and with Guru's Grace we have been able to do intense sadhana to purify the physical body, the astral body, and the causal body. As I mentioned before, all asanas, pranayama, bandhas and mudras end in Kevala kumbhaka, in Unmani avastha (the natural state). The natural state is that state where there is no duality. Kevala umbhaka means suspension of prana in the Ida and Pingala so that the prana moves only in the Sushumna.

It took innumerable births for you to reach this stage. Do not stop your practices now. Lead a moderate and dedicated life. Do not go too fast and then stop the practices because of kickback. Do not go so slow that you get discouraged from lack of visible progress.

Do not be anxious, constantly thinking of your spiritual progress. There will be ups and downs. It is not a straight path. Be courageous. Climb. There will be so many falls; so many ascents you will have to make; so many ropes to tie. There will be so many camps you have to make: base camp, second camp, third camp, fourth camp, and finally, no camp at all when you are left alone to reach the final summit. Nobody to help you now, you will be there alone. But you are not disheartened as you want to reach the top.

In this very life, seek the summit. Pray. Surrender. Our will needs God's Grace, because our will is only a drop. God's Grace is like the ocean. Our willpower is not sufficient to cross the ocean of samsara. Our effort is like a tiny boat with broken oars crossing the Atlantic Ocean; only God's Grace will see us across the ocean.

You must have dispassion and discrimination. While immersed in the activities of life, it is very difficult to keep dispassion, it is very difficult to keep discrimination. But don't forget your goal. Keep Mount Everest always in view. Always look up. Go up a little bit more each time, till your last breath. Never stop your sadhana, your evolution. Look always up, up, up. Go onwards always. It doesn't matter in which state you are, still you have to climb. Never be satisfied with your progress, with your success, with your mental control, because that same mind is waiting for you.

There will be rocks, snow, glaciers, so you will have to go to the right and to the left, but still you will trip and fall. Always pray to God, "Help me, let me not fall again." Prostrate. Surrender to Him. Your effort alone is not sufficient. You can't see the hidden pitfalls. But with surrender, and with your straightforward and honest practice of yama and niyama, you will reach the goal.

May the Lord Bless you with success and liberation in this very lifetime.

Swami Vishnudevananda

GLOSSARY
OF SANSKRIT TERMS
[Guide to pronunciation is within brackets]

Abhiniveśa: Earnest desire; ardent longing; perseverance; clinging to life.

Ācamana: Sipping of water to purify before religious ceremonies.

Ācārya: Spiritual guide or perceptor.

Ādhibhautika: Suffering caused by animals; bee strings, snake bites, attacks by lions, amoebic dysentery, etc.

Ādhidaivika: Suffering caused by planetary influences; natural disasters such as earthquakes, floods, windstorms, etc.

Ādhyātmika: Physical (bodily) and mental suffering.

Adhikārī: A sincere spiritual aspirant with proper qualifications.

Ādinātha: The first Lord; a name for Śiva.

Advaita: Non-dualistic philosophy, Non-dualism.

Aham: Sense of 'I' or ego.

Ahimsā: Non-violence in thought, word and deed, mercy. This is one of the Yamas (restrictions) of Rāja Yoga.

Ājñā: The sixth cakra; the centre of spiritual energy between the two eyebrows; the "third eye."

Ākāśa: Space; either.

Anāhata: (1) The fourth cakra, corresponding to the heart plexus. (2) Astral, "unstruck" or soundless sounds. Mystical sound which is heard by yogīs.

Ānanda: Bliss, joy, infinite happiness.

Ananta: (1) The thousand-headed serpent on which Viṣṇu reclines. (2) Endless.

Aṇimā: One of the eight major siddhis; the power to assume a minute form.

Antaḥkaraṇa: The inner instrument. The ego or "self arrogating" principle.

Anuloma Viloma: Alternate nostril breathing.

Apāna: The downward-moving manifestation of Prāṇa, controls excretion and all the functions of the lumbar region of the autonomic nervous system. The seat of apāna is in the anus; its color is a mixture of red and white.

Aparigraha: Non-receiving of gifts (bribes). One of the Yamas (restrictions) of Rāja Yoga.

Asamprajñāta samādhi: Superconscious state where the mind is totally annihilated, and Reality is experienced. Having no consciousness of the triad; knower, knowledge and the known. The highest state of Rāja Yoga.

Āsana: Posture or position. Poses for meditation and/or body control.

Aṣṭāṅga: Eight limbed; Aṣṭāṅga Yoga is another name for Rāja Yoga.

Āśrama: Hermitage or monastry.

Aśvinī mudrā: A practice to help control the sex urge; while sitting in water, contract and release the anal sphincter muscles, trying to draw the prāṇa upwards.

Asmitā: Egoism.

Asteya: Non-stealing. This is one of the Yamas (restrictions) of Rāja Yoga.

Āstikya: Belief in God.

Asura: A demon; a being yof darkness.

Ātman: The individual self; the Self.

Avatāra: An incarnation of God in physical form.

Avidyā: Ignorance.

Bandha: Muscular locks applied by yogīs during certain breathing exercises. These are essential in advanced prāṇāyāma, in order to direct and unite the prāṇa and apāna. For further details, see pages 247-250 in *Complete Illustrated Book of Yoga.*

Basti: Lower colon irrigation/cleansing; one of the Ṣaṭ kriyās.

Bhadrāsana: Described in *Haṭha Yoga Pradīpīkā*, chapter 1, vs 53,54; in *Complete Illustrated Book of Yoga*, see plates 116-117; also known as Gorakṣana.

Bhagavad Gītā: Literally translated as the "Song of God," this is one of the great Hindu sacred books.

Bhāgavatam: The Purāṇa (a category of Hindu sacred texts) dealing with the exploits and incarnations of Viṣṇu.

Bhakta: A spiritual devotee. A follower of the path of Bhakti Yoga.

Bhakti Yoga: The path of devotion.

Bhārata-varṣa: India

Bhastrika: An important, slightly advanced prāṇāyāma. Forcefully inhaling and exhaling like the bellows of a blacksmith. It has the effect of neither heating nor cooling, but of bringing the body into balance. See chapter 2, vs 59-67.

Bhāva smādhi: The highest state of Bhakti Yoga in which the devotee has the attitude of identification with the Divine.

Bhogārāmās: Those people who indulge in pleasure and live for enjoyment.

Bīja mantra: The seed or root syllable which contains a specific power.

Bindu: The dot or point, which is the center of the nucleus. Static energy.

Brahmā: The Creator in the Hindu trinity of Brahmā, Viṣṇu and Śiva not be confused with Brahman (the Absolute).

Brahmacārī: A student; one who practices brahmacarya.

Brahmacarya: Celibacy, or control of the sexual energy. This is one of the Yamas (restrictions) of Rāja Yoga.

Brahma granthi: First knot in the Suṣumnā, located at the Mūlādhāra cakra.

Brahman: The Absolute Reality.

Brahma-nāḍī: Another name for Suṣumnā.

Brahmarandhra: Literal meaning is "Brahma's Canal" or "the entry to Brahman," it is located in the center of the Suṣumnā nāḍī. Opening of the skull; head fontanelle.

Bhramarī: A minor prāṇāyāma; a light variety of breathing exercise See chapter 2, vs 68.

Brahmavariṣṭha: A yogī who has attained the seventh, and highest, state of Jñāna, who remains in a state of perpetual samādhi.

Brahmavit: Knower of Brahman; a sādhaka who has reached the Sattvāpatti (fourth) stage of Jnāna.

Brahmavivara: A Yogī who has reached the Asaṃśakti (fifth) stage of Jñāna.

Brahmavidyā: The science of Brahman.

Buddhi: Intellect.

Caitanya: Pure consciousness.

Cakra: The astral centres, located in the Suṣumnā.

Cit: Consciousness.

Citta: The subconscious mind.

Crore: Ten million; one hundred lakhs.

Dāna: Giving of charity.

Deva: A shining being; a celestial being.

Dhāraṇā: Concentration; the sixth limb of Rāja Yoga.

Dharma: Righteous conduct.

Dhātus: The tissues of the body: skin, flesh, bones, marrow, fat, and semen.

Dhauti: Cleansing of the upper digestive tract (i.e. mouth,

oesophagus and stomach); one of the Ṣaṭ kriyās.

Dhanurāsana: The "Bow" Pose, *Haṭha Yoga Pradīpīkā*, chapter 1, vs 25.

Dhyāna: Meditation; the seventh limb of Rāja Yoga.

Dṛṣṭi: Seeing, viewing. Seeing with the mental eye.

Dveṣa: Repulsion; hatred.

Gajakaraṇī: Also known as Kuñja kriyā or Gaja karma. In this form of Dhauti, a large quantity of lukewarm water is drunk and then vomitted up.

Gandhara: One of the ten major nāḍīs.

Griman: One of the eight major siddhis; the power to become very heavy.

Gāyatrī: One of the most sacred Vedic mantras; goddess.

Gītā: Usually referring to Bhagavad Gītā.

Gomukhāsana: "Cow's Head Pose," described in *Haṭha Yoga Pradīpīkā,* chapter 1, vs 20; in *Complete Illustrated Book of Yoga*, see plate 122.

Gorakṣāsana: Another name for Bhadrāsana.

Granthi: Three knots, or protective blockages in the Suṣumnā. Their purpose is to block the upward flow of prāṇa. They function as fuses or circuit breakers to protect the practitioner from an energy overload. The knots will only open when sufficient purification and strengthening has taken place.

Gṛhastha: A householder, or married person.

Guṇa: Quality or attribute. One of three qualities of Nature (or Prakṛti): Sattva, Rajas and Tamas.

Guptāsana: See chapter 1, vs 37; also known as Muktāsan.

Guru: Teacher or perceptor.

Gurukula: The system by which the student went to live in the teacher's āśrama. The perceptor's hermitage.

Guruparaṃparā: The guru-disciple lineage.

Haṭha Yoga: The path of Yoga giving first attention to the

physical body, which is a vehicle for the spirit; preference is given to the mobilization of the body and the control of the vital breath. It can be divided as follows:

1. Internal and external purification of the physical body (Kriyās).

2. Practice of Āsanas (physical exercises).

3. Practice of Mudrās and Bandhas.

4. Prāṇāyāma: Control of the vital energy.

5. Pratyāhāra: Withdrawing the mental energy from external stimulation.

6. Dhāraṇā: Concentration.

7. Dhyāna: Meditation.

8. Samādhi: Superconscious state, when the individual consciousness, or ego, merges with the Supreme Consciousness, or Brahman.

Hiraṇyagarbha: Literally meaning "born of a golden egg." Cosmic mind.

Iḍā: The nāḍī to the left of the Suṣumnā. Its nature is intuitive, holistic, inner-directed, emotional, subjective, feminine, cool.

Indriya: Sense organ. There are 5 Jñāna indriyas (organs of knowledge: taste, touch, smell, sight and hearing) and 5 Karma indriyas (organs of action: hands, feet, tongue, anus, and genitals).

Īśvara: God in the form of the chosen deity. Brahman as filtered through the Upādhīs.

Īśvarapraṇidhāna: Surrender to the will of God or surrender of the ego. One of the Niyamas (prescribed observances) of Rāja Yoga).

Īṣitā: One of the eight major siddhis; the power to shape anything as desired.

Jāgrat: The awake state of consciousness.

Jālandhara bandha: The chin lock, forcing the prāṇa

downward. The chin is brought down to touch the Kaṇṭha kūpa (sternal notch).

Jala neti: One of the Ṣaṭ kriyās; water is poured into one nostril and comes out by the other (or through the mouth).

Jambu-dvīpa: Indian sub-continent.

Janaka: Name of a royal sage.

Japa: Repetition of Mantras of God's name.

Jihvā bandha: The tongue lock, to be done with Jālandhara bandha. The top of the tongue is flat against the roof of the mouth and drawn back as much as possible.

Jīvātman: The individual self.

Jīvanmukti: Self-realization while living.

Jñāna: Knowledge; wisdom.

Jñāna Yoga: The intellectual or philosophical path.

Jñānī: A sage or wise person.

Jyoti: Light.

Kaivalya: Absoluteness. Isolated freedom; state of absolute independence.

Kalā: The transcendental wave; energy. A ray, digit of manifestation.

Kali-yuga: The last of the four Hindu time cycles; the present is the "Iron Age."

Kanda: The place near the navel where the nāḍīs unite and separate. It is described as soft, white and egg-like, covered by membraneous membranes. From the kanda spring the 72,000 nāḍīs. It is like a battery, with wires (nāḍīs) going to all parts of the (astral) body. Some yogīs equate the kanda with the preineum, the space between the two legs.

Kapālabhāti: Literally translated as "shining skull." Breathing exercise for cleansing the respiratory system. One of the Ṣaṭ kriyās (six cleansing exercises).

Karma: Action; the law of action and reaction, or cause and effect.

Kevala kumbhaka: Absolute or natural retention (with no effort).

Khecharī mudrā: See chapter 3, vs 33-43.

Kīrtana: Singing the Lord's name.

Kleśas: Pain, anguish, suffering, distress, trouble.

Kriyā: A cleansing or purificatory exercise.

Kukkuṭāsana: The "Cock" pose, described in *Haṭha Yoga Pradīpikā,* chapter 1, vs 23;

Kumbhaka: Retention of breath.

Kuṇḍalinī: Serpent Power; the primordial cosmic energy located in the individual.

Kuñja kriyā: In this form of Dhauti, a large quantity of lukewarm water is drunk and then vomited up.

Laghiman: One of the eight major siddhis; the power to become very light.

Lakh: One hundred thousand (100,000).

Laya: Absorption of mind. Merging; dissolution.

Liṅga: Symbol of Śiva, representing the unmanifested.

Lotus Pose: Padmāsana; see chapter 1, vs 21, 23, 34, 44-49.

Madhyamārga: Literally translated as "the middle path," it is usually used to refer to the Suṣumnā.

Mahā bandha: See chapter 3, vs 19-24.

Mahā mudrā: See chapter 3, vs 14-18.

Mahāpatha: "The great road"; refers to the Suṣumnā.

Mahātmā: A great soul; a saint.

Mahā vedha: See chapter 3, vs 25-29.

Maheśvara: The Great Lord; a name for Śiva.

Mahiman: One of the eight major siddhis; the power to assume a large form.

Mala: An impurity of the mind: lust, anger, greed etc.

Mālā: A garland or necklace.

Manonmanī Avasthā: The state attained when the prāṇa enters the Suṣumnā.

Manana: Thinking, reflection, cogitation; an inference arrived at by reasoning. This is an aspect of Svādhyāya (study).

Manas: Mind.

Maṇipūra Cakra: The third cakra, located in the nābhi (navel) in the Suṣumnā.

Maraṇa: (1) Death, one of the 5 avasthās (states of consciousness). (2) Killing, destruction.

Maṭha or maṭh: A cottage; a small āśrama or monastery.

Mātrā: An ancient measure of time; approximately 3 seconds.

Matsyendrāsana: Spinal Twist. Described in *Hatha Yoga Pradīpīkā,* chapter 1, vs 30; in *Complete Illustrated Book of Yoga,* see plate 101-104.

Mayūrāsana: The "Peacock" pose. Described in *Hatha Yoga Pradīpīkā,* chapter 1, vs 30, in *Complete Illustrated Book of Yoga,* plates 105-109.

Meru: The fabulous mountain at the centre of the universe, around which all the planets are said to revolve. The central bead in a mālā, or rosary.

Mokṣa: Liberation.

Moorcha or Mūrcha: (1) A minor prāṇāyāma; a light variety of yogic breathing. (2) Trance state, one of the 5 avasthās (states of consciousness). See chapter 2, vs 99.

Mudrā: (1) Hatha Yoga exercise, usually used with bandhas, whose purpose is to seal the union to prāṇa-apāna. (2) In Indian dance: hand gestures.

Muktāsana: Also known as Guptāsana; see chapter 1, vs 37.

Mukti: Emancipation.

Mūlādhāra cakra: The first, or lowest, center of spiritual energy located at the base of the spine.

Mumukṣutva: A burning desire for liberation and an intense striving to attain it. One of the four necessary qualifications of a serious student of yoga.

Muni: An ascetic.

Nāda: Mystical sound. Sound or energy wave. Nāda and bindu are represented by Śiva and Śakti.

Nāḍī: An astral nerve. The Sanskrit term equivalent to the "meridians" of acupuncture.

Narakas: Hells; places of purification after death.

Nārāyaṇa: Viṣṇu, the preserver of the universe.

Naṭarāja: The dancing Lord Śiva.

Nauli: Manipulation and churning of the abdomen; one of the Ṣaṭ kriyās (six cleansing exercises).

Neelkaṇṭha or Nīlakaṇṭha: "Blue-throated"; a name for Śiva.

Neti: Cleansing of the upper respiratory tract (i.e. nose, nasal passages, sinuses); one of the Ṣaṭ Kriyās (six cleansing exercises).

Nirālamba: Without support.

Nididhyāsana: Profound and deep meditation.

Nirañjana: The pure consciousness which is free of all qualities or attributes.

Nirvikalpa samādhi: The superconscious state where the mental modifications cease to exist. The term used in Jñāna Yoga.

Niyama: Religious observances, such as cleanliness, contentment, austerity, study and worship of God; the second limb of Rāja Yoga.

Om: The sacred monosyllable which symbolizes the Absolute.

Om Namaḥ Śivāya: The Pañcakṣara (five-littered) mantra of Lord Śiva.

Om Namo Nārāyaṇāya: The mantra of Viṣṇu.

Padma: Lotus.

Padmāsana: See Lotus Pose.

Pāpa: Vice, evil.

Parabrahman: The Absolute.

Paramātman: The Supreme Self.

Parārthabhāvinī: The sixth stage of Jñāna, where external things do not appear to exist.

Paraśakti: The highest energy; Kuṇḍalinī. The Supreme Goddess.

Pārvatī: Lord Śiva's consort.

Paścimatāsana: The Forward Bend pose, described in *Hatha Yoga Pradīpīkā,* chapter 1, vs 28-29. In *Complete Illustrated Book of Yoga,* see plates 55-57.

Patañjali: Author of the Rāja Yoga Sūtras.

Piṅgalā: The nāḍī to the right side of the Suṣumnā; its nature is aggressive, logical, sequential, analytical, outer-directed, rational, objective, hot, masculine, directing mathematical and verbal activities.

Plāvinī: A minor prāṇāyāma; a light variety of yogic breathing exercise. See chapter 2, vs 70.

Prakāmya: One of the eight major siddhis; the power to obtain whatever is desired.

Prāṇa: The vital force. Although prāṇa is one, it takes five major forms (i.e. prāṇa, apāna, samāna, udāna and vyāna). Prāṇa governs the cervical portion of the autonomic nervous system, the verbal mechanism and the vocal apparatus, the respiratory system and the movements of the gullet. The seat of prāṇa is in the heart.

Praṇava: The sacred monosyllable OM.

Prāṇāyāma: The science of breath control. Control of the Prāṇa (vital energy).

Prāpti: One of the eight major siddhis; the power to reach distant objects.

Prārabdha: The karma which has started to fructify in this lifetime.

Pratyāhāra: Abstraction of the senses; withdrawal of the mental energy from the senses. The fifth step of Rāja Yoga.

Puṇya: Merit.

Pūraka: Inhalation of breath.

Purāṇa: Eighteen scriptures of Hindu myths and legends. Sacred works dealing with the doctrines of creation, etc.

Puruṣa: The Supreme Being.

Rāga: (1) Attachment. (2) A tune.

Rāja Yoga: The kingly science; the eight-limbed Yoga of Maharṣi Patañjali.

Rajas: Activity, passion, stimulation, restlessness.

Rajoguṇa: The quality of Rajas, or activity; one of its symptoms is fickleness of mind.

Rāmāyaṇa: The Hindu epic dealing with the life of Śrī Rāma.

Recaka: Exhalation of breath.

Ṛṣi: A seer or sage.

Rudra granthi: The last knot in the Suṣumnā; it is located at the Ājñā cakra.

Sādhaka: A spiritual aspirant; a seeker.

Sādhana: Spiritual practice.

Sahaja: Natural.

Sahasrāra: The seventh or highest cakra; the "thousand-petal lotus." The highest psychic centre wherein the yogī attains union between the individual self and the universal self.

Sahita kumbhaka: The regular retention of breath, either inside or outside of the body.

Samādhi: The Superconsciousness state.

Samāna: One of the five major prāṇas; performs digestion and controls secretions of the digestive system throughout the sympathetic nervous system in the thoracic region. Its seat is in the region of the navel.

Samhitā: Classical texts on Haṭha Yoga include: *Śiva*

Samhitā, Gheraṇḍha Samhitā, Gorakṣa Samhitā.

Samprajñāta samādhi: Contemplation where the consciousness of duality still lingers.

Saṃsāra: The continuous round, or wheel, of births and deaths.

Saṃskāras: Subtle impressions of past lives.

Saṃyama: The simultaneous occurrence of concentration, meditation, and samādhi in a developed yogī.

Sandhyāvandana: Prayers at dawn and dusk.

Saṅkalpa: Thought, imagination.

Sannyāsin: A renunciate; a monk.

Santoṣa: Contentment. One of the Niyamas (prescribed observances) of Rāja Yoga.

Satcidānanda: Existence Absolute, Knowledge Absolute, Bliss Absolute.

Sattva: The quality of purity.

Sattvāpatti: Attainment of the state of purity; fourth state of Jñāna (Knowledge).

Satyam: Truthfulness. This is one of the Yamas (restrictions) of Rāja Yoga.

Śauca: Cleanliness or purity. One of the Niyamas (prescribed observances) of Rāja Yoga.

Śavāsana: The Corpse pose; chapter 1, vs 32. In *Complete Illustrated Book of Yoga,* see plate 146.

Śeṣa: (1) The thousand-headed serpent on which Viṣṇu sleeps. (2) Balance, remainder, what is left.

Ṣaṭ kriyās: The six cleansing exercises, i.e. Neti, Nauli, Dhauti, Basti, Trāṭaka and Kapālabhāti.

Ṣaṭ sampat: The six-fold virtues.

Śakti: Power, energy. Goddess. Female power.

Śakti cālana: An exercise for raising the Kuṇḍalinī.

Śāmbhavī: Pertaining to the auspicious Śambhu, the term

is often used to refer to the Suṣumnā.

Śaṃbhu: Happiness; one who grants prosperity. A name for Śiva.

Ṣaṇmukhī mudrā: Also known as Yoni mudrā. Each ear is closed with the thumb, each eye with the forefinger, the nose with the middle fingers, and the mouth with ring and little fingers.

Śaṅkarācārya: The eighth century philosopher and exponent of Advaita Vedānta. Founder of the Śaṅkarācārya maṭhas.

Śāstras: Sacred texts.

Śūnya: The void; without time or space awareness; having no qualities.

Siddha: One who possesses Siddhis or psychic powers.

Siddhāsana: Many yogīs feel that this is the most important of all the 84 lakh āsanas.

Siddhis: Psychic powers.

Siṃhāsana: The "Lion" Pose, described in *Haṭha Yoga Pradīpīkā,* chapter 1, vs 50-52. In *Complete Illustrated Book of Yoga,* see plate 145.

Śītalī: A minor prāṇāyāma performed with the tongue folded in half; a light breathing exercise which is cooling to the body. See chapter 2, vs 57-58.

Sītkārī: A minor prāṇāyāma performed with the tongue folded back; a light breathing exercise which is cooling to the body. See chapter 2, vs 54-56.

Śiva: The destructive aspect of Godhead, also the Supreme Lord. The bestower of auspiciousness on His devotees.

Śloka: A verse.

Smaraṇa: Remembrance.

Smaśāna: Literally translated as "the burning ground," it is another name for the Suṣumnā.

Smṛti: That which has been remembered. Works of law-givers like Manu which are inferior to the Śruti or revealed scriptures on a point of religious authority.

Soma: Nectar of the moon; divine nectar.

Śrīmad Bhāgvatam: The holy scripture of the Hindus wherein the life and teachings of Kṛṣṇa appear; the incarnations of Viṣṇu and attendant philosophy are explained.

Śravṇa: Listening to spiritual or religious discourse; an aspect of Svādhyāya.

Śruti: Scriptures which are heard.

Śubhecchā: Longing for the Truth; the first stage of Jñāna (Knowledge).

Śūnyapadavī: The great void.

Sūrya: The Sun.

Sūryabheda: An advanced prāṇāyāma which increases the heat in the body; see chapter 2, vs 48-50.

Suṣumnā: The central nāḍī, or astral nerve, which runs through the spinal cord.

Suṣupti: Deep sleep, one of the 5 avasthās (states of consciousness).

Sūtra neti: One of the Ṣaṭ kriyās in which a string (or catheter) is passed through the nose and comes out the mouth, with the purpose of cleansing the nasal passage.

Svādhyāya: Study of scriptures, or spiritual books. One of the Niyamas (prescribed observances) of Rāja Yoga.

Svapna: Dream state of consciousness.

Svarūpa: Essence; the essential nature of Brahman.

Svastikāsana: An important sitting pose, described in *Haṭha Yoga Pradīpīkā,* chapter 1, vs 19. In *Complete Illustrated Book of Yoga,* see plates 17-18.

Svātmārāma: Author of *Haṭha Yoga Pradīpīkā;* the literal translation of his name is "he who is sporting in his own Ātman."

Tamas: The quality (guṇa) of darkness, inertia and infatuation.

Tāmasika: Impure, rotten (with reference to food), lazy, dull.

Tantras: A path of Sādhana laying great stress upon repetition of Mantra and other esoteric meditations.

Tanumānasā: Fading out of the mind; the third stage of Jñāna (Knowledge).

Tapas: Austerities, or penances. One of the Niyamas (prescribed observances) of Rāja Yoga.

Tattva: Principle; the Supreme Principle or Brahman.

Trāṭaka: Steady gazing with the purpose of cleansing and strengthening the eyes and frontal region. It also improves concentration. One of the Ṣaṭ Kriyās.

Turīya: (1) The state wherein the yogī sees God everywhere (2) The state of superconsciousness, the fourth state transcending the waking, dreaming and deep sleep states.

Udāna: One of the five major prāṇas with its seat in the throat, Udāna controls the swallowing of food and the duties which take the individual to sleep. Its realm of activity is above the larynx and it controls all the automatic functions of the autonomic nervous system that take place in the skull. Udāna also functions as a psychic force that separates the astral body from the physical body at the time of death.

Uḍḍiyāna bandha: One of the three most important bandhas, in which the belly is contracted after exhalation.

Ujjāyī: An advanced prāṇāyāma; see chapter 2, vs 51-53.

Unmanī Avasthā: Haṭha Yoga samādhi through control of the prāṇa.

Upīdhi: Limiting adjunct.

Uttāna Kūrmāsana: The "Lifted Tortoise" pose, described in chapter 1, vs 24. In *Complete Illustrated Book of Yoga*, see plate 131. Also known as Garbhāsana (foetus pose).

Uttarakāśi: Himalayan region where Swami Vishnu-devānanda did his period of intensive sādhana.

Vairāgya: Dispassion. Perfect indifference to any object of

desire of earthly life.

Vajrāsana: Kneeling pose; Energy pose.

Vajroli mudrā: A practice which is not followed in sāttvika sādhana.

Vāsanās: Subtle desires.

Vaśitva: One of the eight major siddhis; the power to control anything.

Vāyu: Air; gaseous matter.

Vedānta: Literal meaning is "the end of the Vedas." The school of thought based primarily on the Upaniṣads. The philosophy of Oneness; the end (goal) of Knowledge.

Vedas: The sacred texts of the Hindus containing the Upaniṣads.

Veeṇā (sometimes spelt Vīṇā): An ancient stringed musical instrument.

Vicāraṇā: Right inquiry; the second stage of Jñāna (Knowledge).

Vidyā: Knowledge, science, art.

Viparīta karaṇī: Literal translation is "Topsy turvy" pose; see chapter 3, vs 79-82.

Vīrāsana: Also known as Padmāsana; chapter 1, vs 21.

Viṣṇu granthi: The second knot in the Suṣumnā, located at the Maṇipura cakra.

Vismṛti: Forgetfulness.

Viśuddha: The fifth cakra, located at the throat.

Viveka: Discrimination between what is permanent and impermanent.

Viveka Cūḍāmaṇi: (Crest Jewel of Discrimination) Śaṅkarācārya's masterpiece of Vedāntic philosophy.

Vrata: Vow; religious observance.

Vṛtti: Thought wave; a wave on the mind-lake. Mental modifiction.

Vyāna: One of the five major prāṇas, Vyāna performs the

circulation of blood. It controls the voluntary and involuntary movements of the muscles, joints and surrounding structures. Vyāna also helps to keep the body in an erect position by generating unconscious reflexes along the spinal cord; it is all-pervading and moves throughout the entire body.

Vyomacakra: Another name for Khecharī mudrā.

Yama: (1) Ethics, restrictions; the first limb of Rāja Yoga. Internal purification through moral training. (2) Death (Time). The Lord of Death. (3) A three-hour period.

Yoga Vāsiṣṭha: An important scripture on Advaita Vedānta philosophy, written in the form of conversation between Rāma and his guru Vasiṣṭha.

ASHRAMS AND CENTRES

Sivananda Ashram Yoga Camp
673, 8th Avenue Val Morin
Quebec JOT 2RO, Canada
Tel : +1.819.322.3226
e-mail: HQ@sivananda.org

Sivananda AshramYoga Ranch
P.O. Box 195, Budd Road
Woodbourne, NY 12788, U.S.A.
Tel: +1.845.436.6492
YogaRanch@sivananda.org

Sivananda AshramYoga Retreat
P.O. Box N7550 Paradise Island,
Nassu, BAHAMAS
Tel: +1.242.363.2902
e-mail: Nassau@sivananda.org

Sivananda Yoga Vedanta
Dhanwantari Ashram
P.O.Neyyar Dam
Thiruvananthapuram Dt.
Kerala, 695 572, INDIA
Tel: +91.471.227.3093 / 2703
e-mail: YogaIndia@sivananda.org

Sivananda Ashram Yoga Farm
14651 Ballantree Lane, Comp. 8
Grass Valley, CA 95949, U.S.A.
Tel: +1.530.272.9322
YogaFarm@sivananda.org

Sivananda Yoga Vedanta
Meenakshi Ashram
Kalloothu, Saramthangi Village
Vellayampatti P.O., Palamedu
(via), Madurai Dist. 625 503
Tamil Nadu, INDIA
Tel: +91.94421.90661/2
e-mail: madurai@sivananda.org

Sivananda Kutir
P.O. Netala, Uttar Kashi Dt
(near Siror Bridge) Uttaranchal,
Himalayas, 249 193, INDIA
Tel: +91.1374.224.159
Or +91 9411.330.495

Sivananda Yoga Retreat House
Am Bichlachweg 40A
A-6370 Reith bei Kitzbuhel,
AUSTRIA
Tel: +43.5356.67.404
e-mail: tyrol@sivananda.net

Chateau du Yoga Sivananda
26 Impasse du Bignon
45170 Neuville aux bois,
FRANCE
Tel: +33.2.38.91.88.82
e-mail: orleans@sivanan

CENTRES

Centro Internacional de Yoga
Sivananda; Julian Alvarez 2201
CP 1425 Buenos Aires,
ARGENTINA
Tel: +54.11.4827.9269/9566
BuenosAires@sivananda.org

Sivananda Yoga Vedanta
Zentrum;
Prinz-Eugenstrasse 18
A-1040 Vienna,
AUSTRIA
Tel: +43.1.586.3453
e-mail: Vienna@sivananda.net

Sivananda Yoga Vedanta Centre
5178 St Lawrence Blvd
Montreal, Quebec H2T 1R8,
CANADA
Tel: +1.514.279.3545
e-mail: Montreal@sivananda.org

Sivananda Yoga Vedanta Centre
77 Harbord Street
Toronto, Ontario M5S 1G4,
CANADA
Tel: +1.416.966.9642
e-mail: Toronto@sivananda.org

Centre Sivananda de Yoga
Vedanta
123 Boulevard de Sebastopol
F-75002 Paris,
FRANCE
Tel: +33.1.40.26.77.49
e-mail: Paris@sivananda.net

GERMANY
Sivananda Yoga Vedanta
Zentrum
Steinheilstrasse 1
D-80333 Munich,
GERMANY
Tel: +49.89.52.44.76
e-mail: Munich@sivananda.net

Sivananda Yoga Vedanta
Zentrum
Schmiljanstrasse 24
D-12161 Berlin,
GERMANY
Tel: +49.30.8599.9799
e-mail: Berlin@sivananda.net

Sivananda Yoga Vedanta
Nataraja Centre
A-41 Kailash Colony
New Delhi 110 048,
INDIA
Tel: +91.11.292.40869/30962
e-mail: Delhi@sivananda.org

Sivananda Yoga Vedanta
Dwarka Centre
PSP Pocket, Sector 6 (near DAV
School)
Swami Sivananda Marg
Dwarka,
New Delhi,
INDIA
Tel: 91 11 64568526
e-mail: Dwarka@sivananda.org

Sivananda Yoga Vedanta Centre
House No. 18, TC 36/1238
Subhash Nagar, Vallakkadavu
PO, Perunthanni, Trivandrum,
Kerala, 695 008,
INDIA
Tel: + 91.471.245.1398 / 245.0942
Trivandrum@sivananda.org

Sivananda Yoga Vedanta Centre
3/655 (Plot No. 131) Kaveri
Nagar
Kuppam Road, Kottivakkam
Chennai 600 041,
INDIA
Tel: +91.44.2451.1626
OR +91.44 2451.2546
e-mail: Chennai@sivananda.org

Sivananda Yoga Vedanta Centre
Plot # 23, Dr Sathar Road
Anna nagar, Madurai 625 025
Tamil Nadu,
INDIA
Tel: +91.452.252.1170
maduraicentre@sivananda.org

Sivananda Yoga Vedanta Centre
6 Lateris St
Tel Aviv 64166,
ISRAEL
Tel: +972.3.691.6793
e-mail: TelAviv@sivananda.org

Centro Yoga Vedanta Sivananda
Roma
via Oreste Tommasini, 7
00162 Rome
ITALY
Tel: +39 06 4549 6529
roma@sivananda.org

Centro de Yoga Sivananda Vedanta
Calle Eraso 4
E-28028 Madrid,
SPAIN
Tel: +34.91.361.5150
e-mail: Madrid@sivananda.net

Centre Sivananda de Yoga
Vedanta
1 Rue des Minoteries
CH-1205 Geneva,
SWITZERLAND
Tel: +41.22.328.03.28
E-mail: Geneva@sivananda.net

Sivananda Yoga Vedanta Centre
51 Felsham Road
London SW15 1AZ
UNITED KINGDOM
Tel: +44.20.8780.0160
e-mail: London@sivananda.net

Sivananda Yoga Vedanta Center
1246 Bryn Mawr
Chicago, IL 60660,
USA
Tel: +1.773.878.7771
e-mail: Chicago@sivananda.org

Sivananda Yoga Vedanta Center
243 West 24th Street
New York, NY 10011,
USA
Tel: +1.212.255.4560
e-mail: NewYork@sivananda.org

Sivananda Yoga Vedanta Center
1200 Arguello Blvd
San Francisco, CA 94122,
USA
Tel: +1.415.681.2731
SanFrancisco@sivananda.org

Sivananda Yoga Vedanta Center
13325 Beach Avenue
Marina del Rey, CA 90292,
USA
Tel: +1.310.822.9642
LosAngeles@sivananda.org

Asociacion de Yoga Sivananda
Acevedo Diaz 1523
11200 Montevideo,
URUGUAY
Tel: +598.2.401.09.29 / 401.66.85
Montevideo@sivananda.org